Eastern European Beauty Secrets and Skin Care Techniques

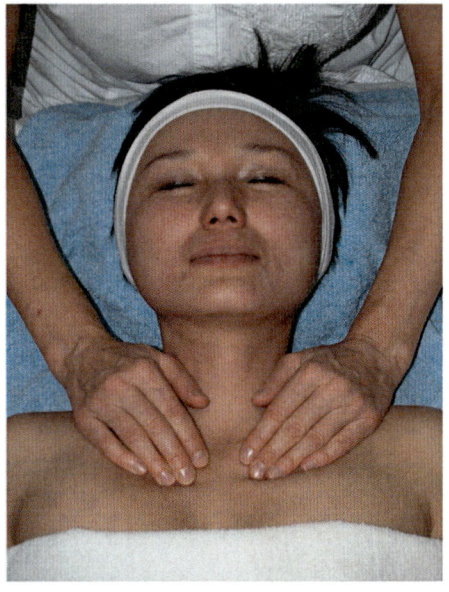

A Practical Manual for Skin Care Professionals

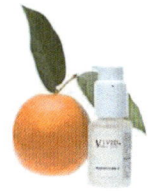

Svetlana Ferguson

Eastern European Beauty Secrets and Skin Care Techniques

By Svetlana Ferguson

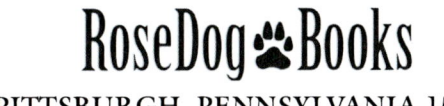

PITTSBURGH, PENNSYLVANIA 15222

The contents of this work including, but not limited to, the accuracy of events, people, and places depicted; opinions expressed; permission to use previously published materials included; and any advice given or actions advocated are solely the responsibility of the author, who assumes all liability for said work and indemnifies the publisher against any claims stemming from publication of the work.

All Rights Reserved
Copyright © 2011 by Svetlana Ferguson

No part of this book may be reproduced or transmitted, downloaded, distributed, reverse engineered, or stored in or introduced into any information storage and retrieval system, in any form or by any means, including photocopying and recording, whether electronic or mechanical, now known or hereinafter invented without permission in writing from the publisher.

RoseDog Books
701 Smithfield Street
Pittsburgh, PA 15222
Visit our website at *www.rosedogbookstore.com*

ISBN: 978-1-4349-8459-3
eISBN: 978-1-4349-7452-5

DISCLAIMER

No part of this book is for the purpose of the treatment of disease.

The author and publisher assume no liability for such use of this book.

Those who have a disease of the skin or other parts of the body should seek competent medical advice.

The use of any skin care techniques or skin care substances discussed in this book rests on judgment of the reader, and any material represented and discussed herein are for educational purposes only and are not intended as recommendations of the author or publisher.

ACKNOWLEDGMENTS

The are not words that can adequately express the challenge and commitment required for writing a book of this scope and nature. The energy that needed to put all pieces of knowledge together, review, write, and edit a 300 page book is almost impossible without other's help.

I am deeply thankful to my friends and colleagues from Ukraine, especially Lesja Biluk who is high-class dermatologist and successful business owner of two esthetic clinics at Lviv, Ukraine. Special thank you to my dearest friend Oksana Narepeha who is a professor of pediatric dentistry at Lviv State Medical University.

I also want to express my endless gratitude for excellent photography work that has done by photography expert Anna Passalaqua and Jylduz Djunushbekova for being the model for my massage techniques.

And most of all, if is not for my husband and soul mate Andrew Ferguson this book would not have been possible. His perseverance and devotion to completing the project go beyond anything I could hope for.

I am blessed to have these people in my life. Without their help and contribution, this book would be an absolutely unconquerable task.

Table of Contents

Introduction xi

Chapter 1: My Story 1

Chapter 2: Structure and Function of the Human Skin 5

Chapter 3: Common Skin Problems 18

Chapter 4: Acne Vulgaris 48

Chapter 5: Rosacea 67

Chapter 6: Skin Aging 76

Chapter 7: Hyperpigmentation 106

Chapter 8: Microdermabrasion and Chemical Peels 115

Chapter 9: Skin Care for Male Clients 129

Chapter 10: Understanding Cosmetic Ingredients 139

Chapter 11: Professional Ethics and Client
 Consultation 163

Chapter 12: Nutritional Supplements for Common
 Skin Disorders 173

Chapter 13: Building a Successful Business 190

Chapter 14: Advanced Skin Care Technology 201

Conclusion 217

Book References and Resources 219

INTRODUCTION

Having acquired information about the vast differences between North American and European esthetic training programs, in this book, I will reveal the secrets of my professional skin care techniques to help skin care specialists build a successful business. This book will target skin care professionals, who want to expand their knowledge of European skin care techniques, and the general public, both women and men, who want to improve their skin care routine.

My work is the outcome of extensive experience and professional knowledge. With 25 years of experience and a medical certification, I have become an esthetic specialist, and it is my goal to now share my knowledge and professional advice on how to achieve outstanding results with esthetic treatments.

My book contains step-by-step European facial techniques, useful tips on how to conduct a successful and profitable business, a list of effective "do-it-yourself" skin care formulas, and other valuable professional advice based on my extensive experience. This book includes every aspect of European skin care techniques, including a detailed protocol for acne treatment and powerful anti-aging procedures, like microdermabrasion and chemical peels.

As a graduate of Lviv State Medical University in the Ukraine, I have created my own skin care formulations that repeatedly were tested and proven to be effective for acne and age related skin problems. You will find recipes for creams, lotions, masks, herbal infusions, and tinctures contained in this book. In addition, I give a detailed introduction to custom blending techniques of cosmetic preparations.

After immigrating to the United States twelve years ago, I have been performing esthetic services at my skin care salon in Durango, Colorado. Having now become a successful business owner, I want to share my experience on how to build a profitable skin care business, develop a business plan, and conduct business marketing and bookkeeping. My advice to keep business overhead low by preparing your own cosmetics is valuable to any professional in the skin care industry.

In addition, you can learn about advanced skin care technology equipment and how to choose the most effective pieces in order to improve services and increase profit. In the **Chapter 14: Advanced Skin Care Technology** I introduce current medical esthetic trends in the skin care industry and describe in detail the principle of each modality. That same chapter contains a description of all the benefits and disadvantages of new technological tools and devices. My goal is to help skin care professionals make appropriate decisions when selecting equipment what will best fit their goals and needs.

Another important aspect that this book covers is a vast of amount of information that can be of interest to general public as well. Additionally, both women and men can benefit significantly from my professional advice on daily skin care routines. You're just a few pages away from learning all my secrets to younger, healthier skin.

CHAPTER 1: MY STORY

My career as a skin care professional started in 1984 after I graduated from the Lviv State Medical University. I was lucky to find a job as a clinical pharmacist in renowned plastic surgery and dermatology clinic, located in Lviv, West of Ukraine.

My job responsibilities required constant mixing, diluting, and preparing varieties of creams, toners, infusions, masks, and other cosmetic preparations. The plastic surgery and dermatology clinic specialized in treating common skin disorders, such as dermatitis, psoriasis, acne, cystic acne, chloazma (hyper pigmentation), malignant skin tumors, skin aging, and much more. The clinic employed two plastic surgeons, five dermatologists, and ten estheticians all working as a team to treat face and body conditions, including hair loss problems.

The clinic was very busy performing skin care, and majority of its clients were seeking esthetician services. Traditionally, the eastern European population will go visit an esthetician for their skin care needs rather than a medical doctor. Many know that even moderate and severe acne problems can be treated by a good esthetician with great results being achieved.

Working there as a pharmacist, I learned a vast amount of knowledge concerning skin problems, and after six years, I decided to switch my carrier to cosmetology. I took extensive cosmetology courses in Lviv and Moscow and started working in the previous clinic as a cosmetologist. Now, I have to mention that "cosmetologists" in the Ukraine refers to the specialist who is trained in skin care only; they do not perform hair and nail services as it commonly seen in United States. Cosmetologists usually have to have a medical background, such as a nursing degree or other medical certification. This is one of the major differences that I have learned after immigration to United States.

My family and I immigrated to United States in 1997. I was very excited to start my career in the States. I made many attempts to find job as a cosmetologist, but it was impossible to use my medical diploma without additional education. However, I simply could not afford additional education, and I decided to receive my license as an esthetician and open my own business.

With time, I became very successful and was performed well all of the services of an esthetician; facials, microdermabrasions, electrolysis, skin peels, and much more.

I have been practicing esthetics in the United States for twelve years now and the first thing that comes to my attention is the fact that European estheticians are trained more extensively than North American estheticians.

There are major differences in both training requirements and hours. The majority of American cosmetology schools offer a 600-hour training program, which is no more than six months or less. Programs for estheticians are even shorter; commonly only a three months requirements. Cosmetology schools offer superficial esthetic training, since it is combined with hair styling, pedicuring, and manicuring.

In contrast, training in Europe is much longer; sometimes up to 3 years in some European countries. The training is also much more intense. The majority of European esthetic schools offer training programs that last from fifteen to twenty-four months with currilicum requirements including anatomy, physiology, biology, microbiology, cosmetic chemistry, dermatology, physics, some pharmacology, medical ethics, and sanitation. Many of European estheticians are CIDESCO certified. The CIDESCO certification program is recognized as the top of international designation for the committed skin care professionals. Many countries recognize CIDESCO as the highest level of achievement in the field of esthetics.

The esthetician profession differs significantly from hairstylists and nail technicians. The major differences lie in the fact that the esthetician performs a treatment while hairstylists and nail technicians provide a service. Skin professionals perform invasive procedures to improve someone's skin condition, which why estheticians in Europe must earn a medical background to practice as an esthetician.

As a skin care professional you are responsible to be able to do the following:

- Recognize existing skin problems that you are dealing with and suggest appropriate treatments.
- Understand cosmetic ingredients and how they affect the skin.
- Understand main principles of bioelectricity and physics in order to successfully perform procedures like ionophoresis (galvanic current), high frequency, ultrasound massage, and more.
- Use all possible safety and sanitation rules when performing skin care procedures.

I stress the role of sanitation and disinfections while working in the beauty industry, dealing with acne vulgaris skin conditions. One the most important steps in the treatment of is a deep pore extraction. Extraction is invasive procedure that deals with puss and even blood. Proper disinfections require the extensive knowledge of sanitation and sterilization procedures. Estheticians have to always be aware of the danger of spreading bacteria, viruses, and disease, and it is essential that they learn the basics of bacteriology and microbiology to insure their containment.

Another aspect that surprised me is the idea that the American facial is being presented as a relaxation procedure rather than a treatment. It appears that massaging hands and feet with high cost cosmetic product are common practice. An excrete from one of the high-end spas in California reads: "Our facial incorporate hot towel wraps and shoulder and neck massages, rubbing essential oils into the face, neck, and shoulders to insure that relaxation is achieved". I am sure that many people like these kinds of services, but they are hardly a skin treatment!

The United States is a newcomer to the field of skin care, with last decade seeing expansion in the pursuits of skin care treatment. Varieties of advanced esthetic courses are now offered at medical esthetic schools. In some states, estheticians can perform procedures like IPL, chemical peels, mesotherapy, microdermabrasions, radio frequency, and laser treatments only under supervision of a physician.

With all that known, I would like to share my broad experience and knowledge for beginners and experienced professionals alike to increase their options in esthetic treatments. I would like to bridge the gap between European education and domestic esthetic training, and represent this book as a reference to skin care treatments. The cosmetic formulations found in the book were given to me from eastern European estheticians, given as beauty secrets, passed down from generation to generation of estheticians.

One such similar story is that of Raya Laboratories, Inc., in Los Angeles, California. Raya herself was an esthetician, living in the former republic of the USSR. She immigrated to the United States and began working in Los Angeles as an esthetician. She became discouraged when she was unable to find the products that she knew would work for her clients. As a European esthetician she knew a lot of skin care formulas that really worked for certain skin problems. With the help of her family, she started a small-scale skin care product line at home. As time passed, her small skin care line evolved into a state -of- the-art, 75,000 sq. feet cosmetic research, development, and manufacturing facility in North Hollywood, California. Currently, Raya Laboratories manufactures over 200, high-quality products available for all skin types and common skin problems. More information may be found on the company website: www.rayalab.com. She is an extraordinary example of one woman's dream to share her knowledge and build a successful business.

Like Raya, I am not soliciting any of the products in this manual, but I simply want to share my knowledge. I invite you to explore my work and the difference it can make for you. You'll discover:

- How to recognize most common skin disorders
- How to conduct proper client consultation
- How to become a multi-treatment skin care specialist by performing a variety of procedures,
- How to read cosmetic labels and understand basic cosmetic chemistry
- What proper nutrition can do to improve skin conditions
- How to build a thriving esthetic business
- How to keep overhead low by creating in- salon cosmetic preparations
- How to develop professional ethics toward clients and co-workers
- How to make smart investments on new tech skin care equipment

Chapter 2: Structure and Function of the Human Skin

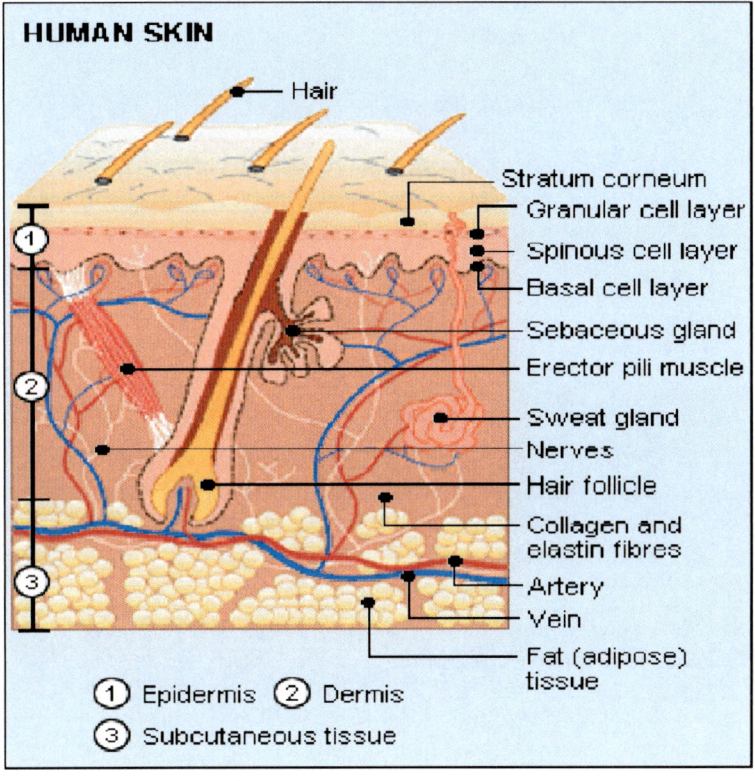

Human skin is a remarkable organ, the body's largest, but it is often take for granted. Most people pay little attention to their skin until a noticeable condition occurs, such as dryness, oiliness, blemishes, or wrinkles. But once they understand how the skin functions, they see the importance of proper care and the quality of skin care products that they use. Therefore, you, as a skin care educator, need to be well versed in explaining to your clients how human skin functions and is structured.

Functions of the Skin

> ➤ It provides protection.

   Skin can protect you from the following:

   - Mechanical impact (pressure and puncture)
   - Thermal impact (heat and cold)
   - Chemical impact (acid, burns)
   - Microorganisms (bacteria, viruses, fungi)
   - UV radiation
     Water loss

> ➤ It aids the immune system.

   Besides providing a biological barrier against microorganisms through its acidic pH-value, the skin is immunologically active through defense mechanisms in the epidermis and dermis. The epidermis and dermis layers of the skin have a large amount of cells (Langerhans cells), which are part of the body's immune system.

> ➤ It regulates body temperature.

   Human body temperature remains stable by evaporation of sweat and water through sweat-producing glands. Another mechanism for rapid cooling is vasodilatation (widening of blood vessels). Heat loss is prevented thought vasoconstriction (narrowing of blood vessels).

> ➤ It is responsible for sensation.

   Nerve endings and receptors located in dermis of the skin are responsible for sensations, such as touch, pain, heat, or cold.

> ➤ It detoxifies.

   Skin cells can detoxify harmful substances though enzymatic processes, with toxins being expelled constantly through sweat glands.

- It produces vitamins.

    Our skin produces Vitamin D through exposure to ultraviolet radiation in sunlight.

- It serves as a communication system.

    The skin has an interactive function of serving as a communication system through paling, blushing, and other expressions, which are regulated by autonomic nervous system.

An adult's skin comprises between 15 and 20 percent of their total body weight. Each square centimeter has 6 million cells, 5,000 sensory points, 100 sweat glands, and 15 sebaceous glands. Skin is being regenerated constantly. The cells migrate upward for about two weeks until they reach the bottom portion of the epidermis, which is the outermost skin layer. The cells spend another two weeks in the epidermis, gradually flattening out and continuing to move toward the surface. Then they die and shed away. Two billion skin cells are shed daily; along with billions of new cells produced. Since the human epidermis is renewed every 15-60 days, proper skin surface nutrition is important to "feed" the cells of the deeper layer of epidermis. Exfoliation will help to remove dry or damaged skin of the outer layer of the epidermis.

Layers of the Skin

The skin has three layers—the epidermis, dermis, and fat layer (also called subcutaneous layer). Each layer performs specific tasks.

Epidermis

The epidermis is the very outer layer of skin. The thickness of the epidermis varies in different skin areas. It is the thinnest on the eyelids (0.05 mm), and it is the thickest on the palms of the hands and soles of the feet soles (0.8 mm).

The epidermis is the relatively thin, tough, outer layer of the skin. Most of the cells in the epidermis are keratinocytes that make the protein named keratin. This is what our hair and nails are made of.

Keratinocytes originate from cells in the deepest layer of the epidermis called the basal layer. New keratinocytes slowly migrate up towards the surface of the epidermis. Once the keratinocytes reach the skin surface, they are gradually shed and are replaced by younger cells pushed up from below.

The epidermis (along with other layers of the skin) also protects the internal organs, muscles, nerves, and blood vessels against trauma. In certain areas of the body that require greater protection (such as the palms of the hands and the soles of the feet), the outer keratin layer of the epidermis (stratum corneum) is much thicker.

Functions of the Epidermis

The epidermis has three principal functions:

- Protecting the body from the environment, particularly the sun
- Preventing excessive water loss from the body
- Protecting the body from infection

Protection from the Environment

The sun produces enormous amounts of heat and light, some of which reaches the earth. Without this heat and light no life could have evolved. Unfortunately, the sun also produces less beneficial rays, which are completely invisible to us, called ultraviolet radiation. This radiation creates high-energy particles, which are called free radicals. Free radical damage may cause wrinkles by activating enzymes (metalloproteinase) that break down collagen, and/or cause cancer by changing the genetic material (RNA and DNA) of the cell. Part of this radiation is reflected by the stratum corneum of the skin's epidermis, and part of it is absorbed by the melanin in the basal layer in the dermis.

Prevention of Water Loss from the Body

Throughout life, our bodies naturally lose water through our skin by constant, gentle evaporation called transepidermal water loss. Preventing excessive water loss is extremely important to the skin itself and to the body as a whole. Water content diminishes as it gets closer to the surface of the skin. It makes up to 70-75% of the weight of the basal layer and 10-15% of the stratum corneum layer.

The stratum corneum layer is an important barrier in controlling moisture loss and environmental damage. When its water content falls below 10%, the skin becomes dry, less flexible, and increasingly prone to damage, breakdown, and infection. The epidermis as a whole is about 35 micrometers thick when dry, but it can swell up to 48 micrometers with full hydration. The thickness depends on the humidity and temperature of the surrounding air as well as our daily water consumption. In fact, drinking six to eight glasses of water a day will not cause water to enter the skin excessively, unless the person is seriously dehydrated. Normal skin is well hydrated naturally. The excess water goes into other tissues of the body and eventually into the bladder.

The most effective way to hydrate the skin is to apply a good moisturizer that supplies water and protects skin from moisture loss.

Protection from Infection

The natural layer of oil-in-water emulsion (oil and sweat), produced in part by the oil glands, is the barrier against invasion by microorganisms, such as bacteria, fungi, and yeast.

The stratum corneum layer of the skin also provides a natural defense against bacteria. White blood cells abundantly found in the stratum corneum layer have the ability to destroy harmful microorganisms invading the epidermis.

The epidermis also contains special defense cells (Langerhans cells), which are located among the keratinocytes. These cells collect invading foreign substances that have found their way into the body, and they take them to white blood cells (lymphocytes) in the lymph glands, where they are neutralized and eventually passed out of the body.

Structure of the Epidermis

The epidermis contains five main layers. They are (from the top layer of skin to the bottom layer of skin):

- Layer #1: Stratum Corneum

    This outermost portion of the epidermis is comprised of dead, flat skin cells that shed about every two weeks. The stratum corneum is waterproof, and when undamaged, it prevents most bacteria, viruses, and other foreign substances from entering the body.

- Layer #2: Stratum Licidum

    The stratum lucidum layer is translucent or transitional layer. This layer is sometimes visible in thick skin, and it performs a transitional role between the stratum corneum and stratum granulosum.

- Layer #3: Stratum Granulosum

    The cells in the stratum granulosum have lost their nuclei, and they are therefore characterized by dark clumps of cytoplasmic material.

Many activities take place in this layer, as keratin and lipid substances are being formed and organized.

- Layer #4: Stratum Spinosum

  Cells that move into the stratum spinosum (also called the prickle cell layer) change from being columnar to polygonal. This layer of epidermis manufactures keratinocytes, which is the main material for the protein keratin.

- Layer #5: Stratum Basale

  The stratum basale is the bottom layer of keratinocytes in the epidermis, and it is responsible for the constant renewal of epidermal cells. This layer contains one row of undifferentiated columnar stem cells that are dividing frequently. Cells divide and push already formed cells into higher layers. As the cells move into the higher layers, they flatten and eventually die.

Scattered throughout the basal layer are cells called melanocytes. These melanocytes produce the pigment melanin, which is one of the main contributors to skin color. Melanin's primary function is to filter out ultraviolet radiation from sunlight that can damage DNA (in the deeper layer of skin), resulting in possible skin cancer.

The basal layer of epidermis also contains Langerhans cells, which are part of the skin's immune system. Although these cells help detect foreign substances and defend the body against infection, they also play a role in the development of skin allergies.

Dermis

The dermis is the middle layer of the skin, located between the epidermis and subcutaneous tissue. It is a thick layer of fibrous and elastic tissue (made mostly of collagen, elastin, and reticular fiber) that gives the skin its flexibility and strength. The dermis varies in thickness, depending on the location. It is about 0.3 mm on the eyelids and close to 3.0 mm on the back.

The dermis is comprised of three types of tissue that are present throughout; collagen, elastin, and fibrillin. Fibrillin is a glycoprotein, which is essential for the formation of elastic fibers, or micro fibrils, that provide strength and flexibility to connective tissue.

The fibroblast is the major cell type of the dermis. These cells produce and secrete procollagen and elastin. Both collagen and elastin are important skin proteins: collagen is responsible to structural support and elastin for resilience of the skin. The proper function of fibroblasts is highly important for overall skin health.

Functions of the Dermis

The primary function of the dermis is to sustain and support the epidermis. Other functions include the following:

- Gives mechanical protection to the body from physical forces
- Provides oxygen and nutrients via tiny blood vessels to the living part of the epidermis
- Removes waste products of cell metabolism in the epidermis via blood vessels
- Provides shape and form to the body by holding all its structures together
- Contributes to skin color. Pale skin contains a little amount of melanin in comparison with dark skin.

Structure of the Dermis

The dermis is subdivided into two main divisions: the deeper reticular layer and the more superficial papillary dermis.

Reticular Layer

The reticular layer of the dermis consists of dense, irregular connective tissue, containing large blood vessels, closely interlaced elastic fibers, and coarse bundles of collagen fibers, arranged in layers parallel to the surface. Surrounding those components is the gel-like ground substance, composed of mucopolysaccharides (primarily hyaluronic acid), chondroitin sulfates, and glycoproteins. The reticular layer is important in giving the skin its overall strength and elasticity, as well as housing other important epithelial-derived structures like glands and hair follicles.

Papillary Dermis

The papillary dermis is thinner, consisting of loose connective tissue, containing capillaries, elastic fibers, reticular fibers, and some collagen. It is named for its fingerlike projections that are called "papillae", which extend toward the epidermis and strengthens the connection between the two layers of skin.

The papillary dermis supplies nutrients to select layers of the epidermis and helps control temperature of the skin surface.

Structure of the dermis also includes nerve endings, sweat glands and oil (sebaceous) glands, hair follicles, and blood vessels. The nerve receptors of the skin sense pain, touch, pressure, and temperature. Some areas of the skin contain more nerve endings than others. For example, the fingertips and bottom of toes contain many nerves and are extremely sensitive to touch.

Sweat glands produce sweat in response to heat and stress. Sweat is composed of water, salt, and other chemicals. As sweat evaporates off the skin, it helps the body to stay cool; thereby, providing thermoregulation of whole body. While the primary function of apocrine (sweat) glands is temperature control, it also plays an important role in excretions of waste products from cells, including ammonia, the product of metabolism lipids and proteins, and other toxins. Certain sweat glands in the armpits and the genital region (apocrine glands) produce thick, oily sweat that contributes to specific body odor.

Sebaceous glands are made of fatty acids, cholesterol, carbohydrates, and triglycerides. They also contain vitamins, hormones, salt, and bactericide substances. For one week, sebaceous glands produce 4-5 gm of sebum, which, combined with sweat, forms the oil-in-water layer. This emulsion has protective and antibacterial properties, therefore, keeping the skin from harmful bacteria. Within hours, sebum undergoes oxygenation and is converted into a substance that can cause skin irritation and inflammation. Harmful bacteria then grow rapidly inside the skin pores, often causing the formation of comedones and inflamed pustules. Indeed, washing your skin is extremely important in order to keep it clean and healthy.

In addition, the sebaceous glands secrete sebum directly into hair follicle to keep hair lubricated and moist.

Many **small blood vessels and hair follicles** are located in the dermis as well. Hair follicles are downward growths into the dermis to produce hair. They are found all over the body except on the palms of the hands, soles of the feet, and the lips. When the body gets cold, the hair stands upright with the help of the arrector pili muscles that attached to the base of the follicle. By this action, the skin's pores close up and keep the warmth in. Therefore, one of the main functions of body hair is thermoregulation. In addition, it plays a sensatory role and provides mechanical and environmental protection.

The blood vessels of the dermis deliver nutrients to the skin and help regulate body temperature. Heat makes the blood vessels enlarge (dilate), allowing large amounts of blood to circulate near the skin surface, where the heat can be released. Cold makes the blood vessels narrow (constrict), thereby, retaining body heat.

The number of nerve endings, sweat glands and sebaceous glands, hair follicles, and blood vessels vary over different areas of the body. The top of the head, for example, has many hair follicles, whereas the soles of the feet have none.

❖ Subcutaneous Tissue or Fat Layer

Below the dermis lies a layer of fat (hypodermis) that helps insulate the body from heat and cold, provides protective padding, and serves as an energy storage area. The fat (adipose tissue) is made of cells called fat cells that are held together by fibrous tissue. The fat layer varies in thickness, from a fraction of an inch on the eyelids to several inches thick on the abdomen and buttocks. The layer of adipose tissue principally serves to insulate the body and to provide mechanical protection against physical shock. The fat cells can also provide a readily available supply of high-energy molecules. The loss of subcutaneous tissue often occurs with age and leads to facial sag and accentuates wrinkles.

Skin Types

To perform proper facial treatment, you have to differentiate what type of skin your client has. Without proper skin analysis, you might choose an inappropriate treatment and offer inaccurate advice for the client's home care. There are five basic skin types. However, a person's facial skin varies at different times throughout their lives, due to aging or other damage. The information below provides general information about five basic skin types.

- Type #1: Normal Skin

    The characteristics of so-called "normal" skin may be summarized as follows:

    - A clear appearance
    - An even color
    - Feels neither tight nor greasy
    - Soft and supple to the touch
    - A high degree of elasticity

    In normal skin, the oil glands produce sebum at a moderate rate, resulting in a balanced state of not too oily and not too dry. Normal skin looks consistently plump, moist, and vibrant, but still requires no less attention than other skin types. Without proper skin care, normal skin can quickly become "abnormal", however. Failure to be attractive or allow abuse by sun, wind, or cold may lead to dry and damaged skin, and ultimately the risk of premature development of lines and wrinkles. Caring for normal skin requires a normal cleaning, toning, and moisturizing.

- Type #2: Dry Skin

    Dry skin is characterized most of all by the sensation of tightness, with the skin feeling rough and scaly and visible lines developing. At its worst, it may look cracked. The problem lies in poor epidermal function and damage of the water/lipid barrier, shown by an increase of transepidermal water loss. Dry skin also is caused by under active or inactive oil glands that do not produce enough sebum to keep the skin naturally lubricated.

    Patches of dry skin may appear on typically normal skin or, sometimes, even on oily skin that has been temporarily dried out by weather extremes (cold, heat, sunlight, wind) or chemicals, such as detergents and solvents. Using harsh commercial soaps or insufficient moisturizers also can cause dry skin. Living in a dry climate can contribute to skin dryness, and you will require intense skin moisturizing along with sufficient water consumption.

    Characteristics of dry skin:

    - Feels tight and irritable
    - Often looks flaky
    - Often develops fine lines around the eyes
    - Tightens after washing with soaps or detergents or prolonged exposure

    Dryness is a significant problem associated with mature skin as hydration ability progressively decreases and the skin's mechanical properties deteriorate along with loss of suppleness and flexibility. An appropriate skin care regime may change the skin condition dramatically. The dryer is the skin, the more hydrating ingredients a moisturizer should contain. For instance, lanolin-based moisturizers will keep skin moist for a substantially long time since lanolin is an excellent water-holding agent. Refer to **Chapter 10: Understanding Cosmetic Ingredients** for a variety of hydrating ingredients.

- Type #3: Sensitive Skin

    Doctors and scientists do not agree completely about what "sensitive skin" is, but generally, it may be considered as skin, which is easily irritated. Sensitive skin is characterized by an inadequate reaction to environmental factors, cosmetic products, water temperature, or other minor irritants.

    Sensitive skin is troublesome for many individuals. It frequently reacts adversely to environmental conditions, such as wind, sun, or extreme temperature changes. This skin type is prone to react to cosmetics containing alcohol, synthetically manufactured oils, essential oils, artificial colors, and fragrances. Consequently, sensitive skin often requires special treatment in order to remain in good condition.

    Another element of sensitive skin is its susceptibility to sunburns. People with a sensitive skin type may experience the following symptoms: rashes and red blotchy patches, itchiness, small breakouts, broken blood vessels, tingling, tightening, and other cutaneous discomforts.

    Sensitive skin also may be associated with a medical condition called atopy or atopic dermatitis, where people have an inherited predisposition to eczema, hay fever, and asthma. Dry atopic skin is vulnerable, especially to winter weather. Protection by generous and frequent application of moisturizer is vital. In addition, sensitive skin benefits greatly from natural gentle skin care products as well as form professional deep moisturizing treatments, including light steaming and hydrating facial masks.

- Type #4: Oily Skin

    Oily skin is caused by sebaceous glands producing too much sebum, resulting in the skin becoming greasy in texture and shiny in appearance with large and clogged pores. This type of skin is a common, particularly in adolescents and young adults, due to hormonal changes drastically increasing sebum production. The extra sebum gives the skin a shiny appearance, especially on the nose and forehead. The epidermis tends to thicken, due to increased keratin production, and the pores become dilated.

    An individual with oily skin may experience the following symptoms:

    - Shiny skin on the forehead, nose, and chin (the T-zone)
    - Thickening of the skin with more visible enlarged pores
    - Pimples, blackheads, whiteheads, and other acne blemishes

- Oily residue apparent in the morning
- Flakiness around the nose area due to dried excess of oils
- Slow to develop discolorations, such as freckles, fine lines, and wrinkles as the skin ages
- Hair become greasy and requires frequent washing

Oily skin requires special products, specifically made for oily skin, with different skin care routine than dry skin. Cleansing should be done with an appropriate cleanser (avoid harsh soaps) at least twice, or sometimes three times, per day. Usage of an oil-control astringent helps to control oil production and keep pores from clogging. Skin with frequent breakouts needs special skin care products containing antibacterial and healing properties.

- <u>Type #5: Mixed Skin or Combination Skin</u>

    Most people have at least two different types of facial skin at any given time. Combination skin, perhaps the most common type of problematic skin, has typical symptoms, including:

    - Forehead, chin, and nose are oily (the T-zone area), but the cheeks and skin around the eyes can range from normal to dry
    - Skin pores are medium in size
    - The skin may be oily along the chin, jaw line, and temples, but dry or normal elsewhere
    - Overall the skin appears normal and healthy, not including those small affected areas that are too oily or dry

Skin care for combination skin should be a dual approach in order to deal with the two different areas of facial skin. More moisture has to be applied the dry part of the face while treating the oily area (T-zone) with a product for oily skin.

Another skin gradation has been used in esthetic practice and that is by skin color and its reaction to sun exposure. The chart below shows the natural pigmentation of skin when exposed to sunlight.

Skin Type	**Unexposed Skin Color**	**Sun Response**
I	white	always burns, never tans
II	white	always burns, tans minimally
III	white	burns minimally, sometimes tans
IV	light brown	burns minimally, always tans well
V	brown	rarely burns, tans darkly (Asian skin)
VI	dark brown	never burns, tans darkly (African skin)

To properly identify the skin type of the person, the esthetician needs to look beyond what can be seen by the naked eye. Dry patches and oily regions of skin that are hardly visible to the naked eye can be seen easily under the Wood's lamp. The Wood's lamp helps the esthetician to analyze skin conditions while observing skin under ultra-violet light. For example, normal and healthy skin shows as blue or white color, dehydrated skin is light violet, oily parts with comedones are yellow or sometimes pink and pigmentation shows as dark brown.

For the past few decades, different manufacturers have developed numerous skin analysis tools and equipment. Skin test devices are designed to make a more accurate skin observation. Proper skin analysis is one of the most important steps for successful treatment, thus it is essential to invest in one of the skin test tools available.

In conclusion, you as a skin expert have to pay keen attention to the skin type to select proper treatment in accordance with the skin needs of your client and be ready to offer a full range of cosmetic products that correspond to their specific skin condition. Based on your professional knowledge, clients should receive qualified advice on how to take care their skin at home.

CHAPTER 3:
COMMON SKIN PROBLEMS

As a skin care professionals, we deal with a variety of skin disorders on a regular basis. Recognition and knowing skin condition is a very important aspect in an esthetician's practice. Persons who are seeking skin care service will rely on your expertise and will expect esthetic professional help.

To work effectively on the skin, the esthetician must be able to recognize various skin disorders and diseases and choose the proper treatment or course of action if it is beyond his or her professional scope. Advanced knowledge of skin imperfections is essential in order to choose the correct type of the treatment that will be most beneficial for the client. However, if a client has a skin condition beyond the scope of the esthetician's responsibility, the esthetician should suggest that their client see a dermatologist. Under no circumstance, should the esthetician ever try to diagnose the condition for client! There are many risks involved in trying to diagnose diseases. Many conditions closely resemble other conditions and require extensive testing to diagnose properly.

Describing most common skin disorders, an esthetician has to be aware of some terminology that is commonly used in esthetics and dermatology:

- *Atrophy:* a thinning/loss of epidermis or dermis
- *Bulla:* large, elevated lesion that contains free liquid (a blister)
- *Crust:* an accumulation of exudates (e.g. blood, puss, serum)
- *Cyst:* a sac containing liquid or a semi-solid, usually found in the dermis
- *Erosion:* a loss of epidermis above the basal layer
- *Excoriations:* crust and erosions due to scratching
- *Fissure:* a slit through the whole thickness of the skin
- *Macule:* small area with change in skin color, but no alternation in skin level
- *Noble:* a palpable solid lesion that usually extends from deeper skin layers to the outer surface
- *Papule:* a solid elevated lesion no more than 1-2 cm
- *Patch:* a macule, but larger
- *Plaque:* a solid, elevated lesion, usually more than 1-2 cm

- *Pustule*: an elevated lesion that contains pus, usually found in the dermis
- *Scale*: excessive layering of keratinocytes on the skin surface
- *Scar*: fibrous tissue formed during wound healing
- *Sclerosis*: a hardening of the skin
- *Ulcer*: a loss of the epidermis and part or all of the dermis, leaving moist lesions
- *Vesicle*: similar to a bulla, but smaller
- *Telangiectasia*: broken capillaries that are visible on the skin surface

Moles

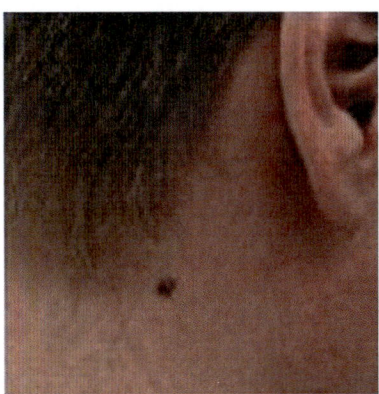
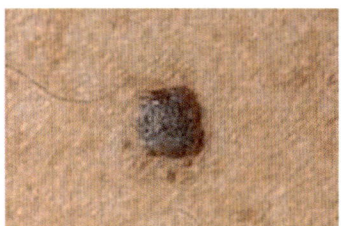

Moles (nevus) are small, usually dark, skin growths that develop from pigment-producing cells in the skin (melanocytes). Moles vary in size from small dots to more than 1 inch (about 2.5 centimeters) in diameter. Almost everyone has a few moles, and many people have large numbers of them. Moles may be flat or raised, smooth or rough (wart like), and they may have hair growing from them. Although they are usually brown or dark brown, some moles are flesh-colored or yellow-brown.

Moles commonly develop in childhood or adolescence; although, in some people, they continue to develop throughout life. Moles respond to changes in hormone levels in women and may first appear during pregnancy. Once formed, moles remain for a lifetime and get less pigmented and more raised under the skin surface with time. In fair-skinned people, moles occur more commonly on sun-exposed areas of the skin. Moles usually are easily recognized by their typical appearance. They do not itch or hurt, and they are not a form of cancer. However, moles sometimes develop into or resemble melanoma, a cancerous growth of melanocytes (see: Melanoma). In fact, many melanomas begin in moles, so a mole that looks suspect should be removed and examined by biopsy.

Some important facts that you should know about moles are:

> - Most people have some moles, but the tendency to develop atypical moles is hereditary.
> - Moles and atypical moles that change drastically should be examine by experienced dermatologist for possible melanoma.
> - Most non-cancerous moles do not require treatment, but moles that are uncomfortable or a cosmetic concern can be removed with a scalpel and local anesthetic.

Melanoma

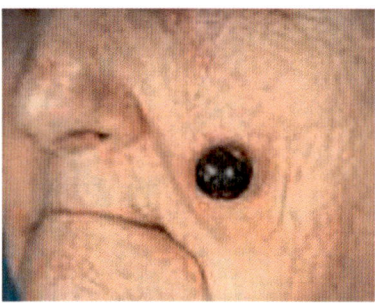
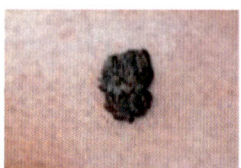

Melanoma is the most serious type of skin cancer. Melanoma may appear on normal skin, or it may begin at a mole (nevi) or other area that has changed in appearance. Often, the first sign of melanoma is a change in the size, shape, color, or feel of the skin. Most melanomas have black or black-blue area. Also, it may be seen as black, abnormal, or "ugly looking". A feeling similar to itching, burning, or pinching may be present as well. The mole may begin to rapidly grow, changing shape and color. The surface of the mole might have lessons that bleeding or oozing.

The most important signs of melanoma are:

- Change in skin color, where color of the skin becomes darker with lighter spots.
- Change in size and shape, characterized by rapid growth
- Change in the surface of the mole and appearance of papillomas, lesions, and broken capillaries
- Increased temperature around the mole and signs of inflammation
- Enlarged regional lymphatic glands

The presence of only one of these signs can be a signal for immediate check up with the doctor. The development of melanoma is related to sun exposure, particularly to sunburns during childhood, and it is most common among people with fair skin, blue or green eyes, and red or blond hair.

Risk factors include the following:

- Family history of melanoma
- Red or blond hair and fair skin
- Presence of multiple birthmarks
- Development of pre cancerous lesions
- Obvious freckling on the upper back
- Three or more blistering sunburns before age 20
- Three or more years spent at an outdoor summer job as a teenager
- High levels of exposure to strong sunlight
- Living in high attitude area

Types of Melanoma

The 4 major types of melanoma are the following:

- Type #1: Superficial Spreading Melanoma
  This is the most common type of skin cancer. It is usually flat and irregular in shape and color, with varying shades of black and brown. It may occur at any age or body site, and it is most common in Caucasians.

- Type #2: Nodular Melanoma
  This usually starts as a raised area that is dark blackish-blue or bluish-red, although some are without color.

- Type #3: Lentigo Maligna Melanoma
  This type usually occurs in the elderly. It is most common in sun-damaged skin on the face, neck, and arms. The abnormal skin areas are usually large, flat, and tan with intermixed areas of brown.

- Type #4: Acral Lentiginous Melanoma
  This is the least common form of melanoma. It usually occurs on the palms, soles, or under the nails, and it is more common in African Americans.

Melanoma can be cured if it is diagnosed and treated early. If melanoma is not removed in its early stages, cancer cells may grow downward from the skin surface and invade healthy tissue. If it spreads to other parts of the body, it can be difficult to control.

If you, as a skin care professional, determine similar symptoms on your client, she or he should be immediately advised to see dermatologist. Your client may not aware of it or may just simply ignoring the visually changes of their mole. Your task as a skin care professional is to acknowledge the present skin disease and refer them to the doctor.

Skin Cancer

Like melanoma, *skin cancer* is very important to be diagnosed and treated in its early stages. Skin cancer is the most prevalent of all types of cancers. It is estimated that more than one million Americans develop skin cancer every year.

Basal Cell Carcinoma

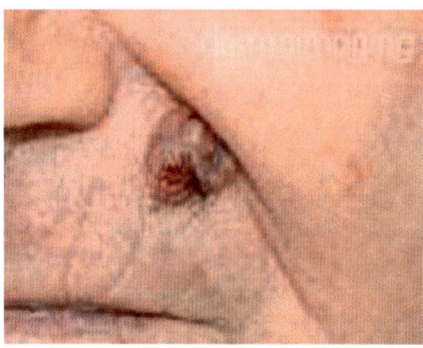
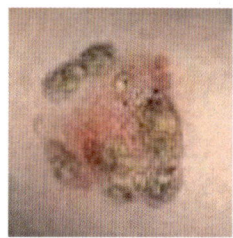

Basal cell carcinoma is the most common form of skin cancer, and it accounts for more than 90% of all skin cancer in the U.S. This cancer almost never spreads (metastasize) to other parts of the body. It can, however, cause damage by growing and invading surrounding tissue.

Basal cell carcinoma appears frequently on the, face, neck, and hands as a small, fleshy bumps, nodules, or a red patch. Other parts of the body may be affected as well. Basal cell carcinomas are frequently found in fair-skinned people and rarely occur in darker skinned people. They usually do not grow quickly. It can take many months or years for one to grow to a diameter of one-half inch. Untreated, the cancer often will begin to bleed, crust over, heal, and repeat the cycle. Untreated, this can extend below the skin to the bone and nerves, causing considerable local damage.

A basal cell carcinoma usually begins as a small, dome-shaped bump, and it is often covered by small, superficial blood vessels called telangiectasias. The texture of such a spot is often shiny and translucent, sometimes referred to as "pearly". It is often hard to tell a basal cell carcinoma from a benign growth like a flesh-colored mole without performing a biopsy. Some basal cell carcinomas contain melanin pigment, making them look dark rather than shiny.

Superficial basal cell carcinomas often appear on the chest or back and look more like patches of raw, dry skin. Basal cell carcinomas grow slowly, taking months or even years to become sizable. Although spreading to other parts of the body (metastasis) is very rare, a basal cell carcinoma can damage and disfigure the eye, ear, or nose if it grows nearby. People with Basal carcinoma must visit the oncologist for regular check-ups for skin disease evaluation.

Risk factors of developing basal cell carcinoma:

- Light-colored skin,
- Sun exposure
- Age

People who have fair skin and are older have higher rates of basal cell carcinoma. About 20% of this skin cancer, however, occurs in areas that are not sun-exposed, such as the chest, back, arms, legs, and scalp. The face, however, remains the most common location for basal cell lesions. Weakening of the immune system, whether by disease or medication, can also promote the risk of developing basal cell carcinoma.

Lipoma

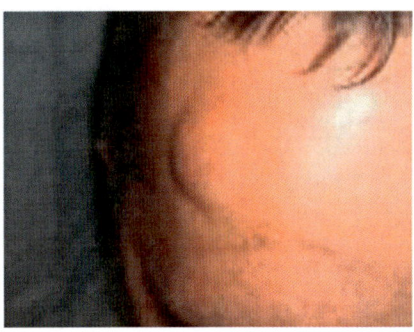
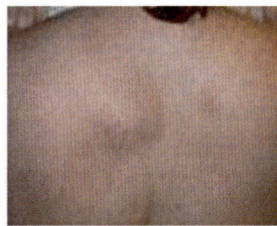

Lipoma is a slow-growing, fatty tumor situated between your skin and the underlying muscle layer. Often, a lipoma is easy to identify because it moves readily with slight finger pressure. It's doughy to touch and usually not tender. Lipomas can occur at any age, but they're most often detected in middle age.

Most often, lipomas remain small — less than 2 inches (5 centimeters) in diameter, but they can grow large, reaching more than 4 inches (10 centimeters) across. Lipomas can be painful if they grow and press on nearby nerves. A lipoma isn't cancer, and it is usually harmless. Treatment generally isn't necessary, but if the lipoma is in a bothersome location or enlarges, surgical removal can be considered.

The exact cause of lipomas isn't clear. Sometimes lipomas are detected after an injury. But it's uncertain whether they're caused by trauma or whether their detection was just incidental. Lipomas also tend to run in families; so genetic factors are likely to play a role in their development.

Dermatofibroma

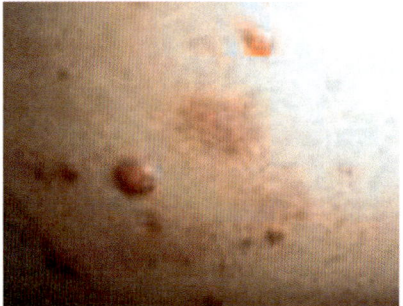

Dermatofibroma is a common cutaneous nodule of unknown etiology that occurs more often in women. It is seen as reddish or yellow-brown nodule with smooth spherical surface. It is most frequently located on the legs, but it can be located on different parts of body as well. Dermatofibroma is a non-cancerous tumor that can be removed only by surgeon.

Epidermal Cysts

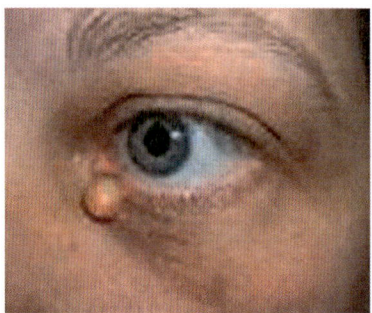 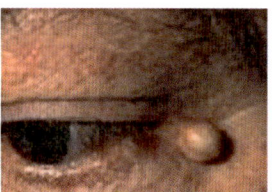

An epidermal cyst is a common slow-growing bump, due to an enlarging sac under the skin that accumulates a cheesy substance that is composed of the skin secretions.

Epidermal cysts, often incorrectly referred to sebaceous cysts, are flesh-colored and range from ½ to 2 inches (about 1 to 5 centimeters) across. They often have an enlarged pore lying on top of them. They can appear anywhere, but they are most common on the back, head, and neck. They tend to be firm and easy to move with the skin. Epidermal cysts are not painful unless they become infected or inflamed.

Large epidermal cysts can be only removed surgically after an anesthetic is injected to numb the area. The thin sac wall must be removed completely or the cyst will grow back. Cysts that have burst under the skin often cause tenderness and swelling and need to be cut open to drain. Tiny cysts that are bothersome and should be drained, and the best idea is to remove them completely.

Xanthelasma

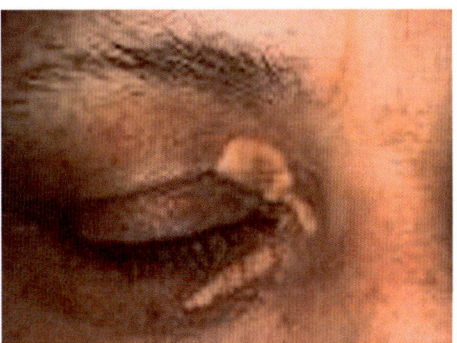
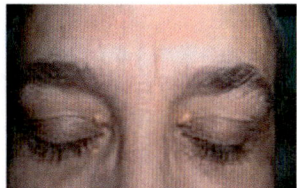

Xanthelasma (or xanthelasma palpebrarum) is a sharply demarcated yellowish collection of cholesterol underneath the skin, usually on or around the eyelids. *Xanthelasma* (or xanthoma) usually occur in people who are suffering from diabetes, liver disease, and/or atheromatous disease (cholesterol building up in arteries). Although not harmful or painful, these minor growths may be disfiguring and should be removed by surgeon. Xanthelasma can be removed with trichloroacetic acid peel or laser or cryotherapy (liquid nitrogen application) Removal can cause scarring and skin pigment changes, but it is unusual after treatment with trichloroacetic acid. Only a licensed medical professional should perform the chemical peel in order to remove xanthoma.

Keratosis

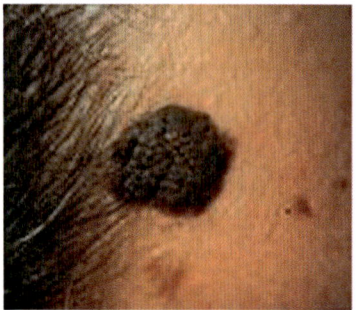

Seborrheic keratosis (Dermatosis Papulosa Nigra) is classically described as looking like someone took clay or a blob of dirt and "stuck" it to the skin. As it develops, some of the basal cell papilomas (seborrheic keratosis) can have a very rough surface with deep pits and fissures, almost like cauliflower being pulled apart. Some seborrheic keratosis doesn't have a rough surface. If they are smooth, they contain tiny bumps that look like seeds that are lighter or darker than the surrounding tissue. These are called horn pearls, and they are actually bits of keratin that develop in a whirling, circular pattern. Sometimes, these horn pearls are best seen with a magnifying glass.

The edge of the dark brown papules is not attached to the underlying skin, making it appear that it could be removed by picking it off with your fingernail. This is because seborrheic keratosis arises from the epidermis, and it does not extend deep into the skin like warts. Seborrheic keratosis may look like warts, but they don't contain the human papilloma viruses that cause warts.

Seborrheic keratosis is usually removed because they itch, they interfere with clothing or jewelry, or they are cosmetically unacceptable. Some people will unintentionally manipulate or "pick at" and cause it to be irritated and inflamed. If irritated enough, the skin around it can become red, and the brown patches can bleed. In this case, the client has to seek immediate medical assistance in order to remove keratosis.

A small seborrheic keratosis can be frozen with liquid nitrogen. Liquid nitrogen works by freezing and destroying the cells but leaving the connective tissue foundation intact. For the most severe cases of seborrheic keratosis, laser treatments or thermo coagulation can be performed by a dermatologist or plastic surgeon.

Keratosis Pilaris

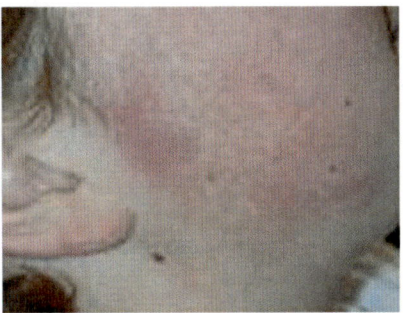

Keratosis pilaris is a very common skin disorder that can be seen in many people of all ages. It is a benign condition that presents as numerous small, rough, red or tan bumps, primarily around hair follicles on the upper arms, legs, buttocks, and sometimes cheeks. Effected areas often look like "goose bumps" or "chicken skin". A majority of people with this skin problem may be unaware that the skin condition has a designated medical term or that it is treatable. In general, this type of keratosis is often cosmetically displeasing, but it is medically completely harmless.

Here are some facts you should know about *keratosis pilaris:*

- ➢ It is seen in patients with very dry skin conditions and atopic dermatitis.
- ➢ Keratosis pilaris is not curable, but it may become less noticeable with time.
- ➢ Keratosis pilaris may spontaneously clear without treatment, but it generally requires ongoing maintenance therapy.

Treating keratosis pilaris with daily moisturizing, gentle exfoliation, and glycolic or lactic acids usually gives successful results. Consider helpful options for keratosis pilaris like chemical peels, microdermabrasion, and facials. There will be more about the treatment of keratosis pilaris in next the following chapter.

Actinic Keratosis

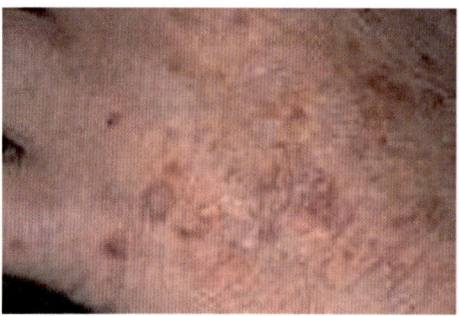

Actinic keratosis (or solar keratosis) is considered the earliest stage in the development of skin cancer. They are small, scaly spots that are most commonly found on the face, ears, neck, lower arms, and the backs of the hands in fair-skinned individuals who have had significant sun exposure.

The effected part of the skin generally measures in size between 2 to 6 millimeters in diameter. The spots are usually reddish in color and often have a white scale on top.

Common locations for actinic keratosis are the face, scalp, back of the neck, upper chest, as well as the tops of the hands and forearms. Men are more likely to develop actinic keratosis on top of their ears.

Actinic keratosis can be treated with cryotherapy (freezing), topical chemotherapy (applying a cream or lotion), chemical peeling, microdermabrasion, laser surgery, curettage, photodynamic therapy (a chemical is applied to the skin prior to exposure to a light source), or other dermatology surgical procedures. Some actinic keratosis may progress to advanced stages that require more extensive treatment. Regular use of sunscreens can help prevent actinic keratosis even after extensive sun damage has already occurred. Estheticians must be very careful with existing problems and advise the client to see dermatologist for further evaluation.

Atopy or Atopic Dermatitis

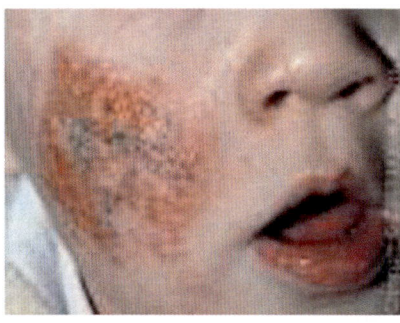
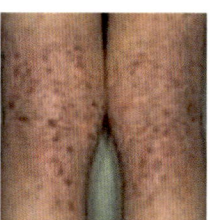

About 20% of the population has the inherited condition called atopy, which can lead to various degrees of dry skin or even eczema. No one knows the precise cause of atopy, except that it has a genetic component: 70% of patients with atopic dermatitis have at least one relative who suffers from eczema, asthma, or hay fever. In childhood, eczema often appears in the creases of the elbows, knees and buttock - the so-called flexural eczema. In adults, eczema tends to form patches on the joins area, especially elbows. Hairline and facial patches can be seen in some individuals. In elderly people, eczema can be associated with poor circulation in the legs: this is known as varicose eczema.

The diagnosis of *atopic dermatitis* is based on the findings of the history and physical examination. Exposure to possible exacerbating factors, such as aeroallergens, irritating chemicals, foods, and emotional stress, should be investigated. The skin lesions observed in atopic dermatitis vary greatly, depending on the severity of inflammation, different stages of healing, chronic scratching, and frequent secondary infections. Acute lesions are papules and vesicles on a background of erythema (redness).

Eczematous skin requires constant moisturizing, and harsh soaps should be avoided. Patients should bathe in warm (not hot) water and use mild, unscented soaps or soap-free cleansers. Liberal amounts of a lubricant or emollient cream should be applied to the skin immediately after bathing. Skin moisturizing lotions should be applied once or twice daily to prevent skin dryness and irritation. Careful use of steroid creams on the body may be helpful, but these products should only be used under medical supervision.

It is essential that estheticians will be able to recognize eczema or dermatitis skin conditions and take right course of action. Please, advise your client to see dermatologist for professional treatment, especially when you notice severe cases of dermatitis. Mild cases of dermatitis can be treated with esthetic procedures. However, procedures like exfoliation and face steaming are strictly prohibited for people with such skin conditions. Below I have posted the symptoms of dermatitis and the protocol for treatment for those with mild to moderate skin problem manifestation.

Contact Dermatitis

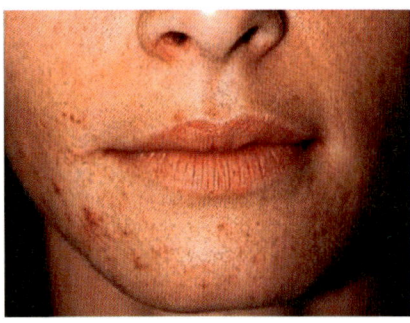
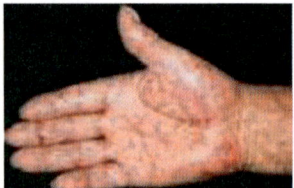

Dermatitis (eczema) is an inflammation of the upper layers of the skin, causing itching, blistering, redness, swelling, blood oozing, scabbing, and scaling. Damaged skin can look slightly swollen with small papules. In more severe cases, it can be seen as many blisters with grayish liquid. In some cases, it looks like a red, itchy rash. The itching is usually severe, but the rash varies from a mild, short-lived redness to severe swelling and large blisters. Most commonly, the rash contains tiny blisters and develops only in areas contacted by the substance. Touching the rash or blister fluid cannot spread contact dermatitis to other people or to other parts of the body that did not make contact with the substance.

Determining the cause of contact dermatitis is not always easy. Dermatitis usually occurs from influence of some physical, biological, and chemical factors directly onto skin. The person's occupation, hobbies, household duties, eating habits, clothing, topical drug use, cosmetics, and household members' activities must be considered.

Physical factors can be trauma, high or low temperature, sunburn and etc. Biological factors can be things like the bites of some bugs or contact with allergenic plants, i.e. poison ivy, poison oak, ragweed, primrose, and thistle. Chemical factors are related to household cleaners, detergents, solvents, cosmetic product, hair dyes, nail polish, deodorants, perfumes, sunscreens, etc...

There is another type of dermatitis related to food intolerance. Some people can have allergic reactions to citrus fruits, gluten, milk, chocolate, or alcohol.

Dermatitis is a very common skin condition. Knowledgeable estheticians should be able recognize the problem and make the right decision as to the treatment, or in severe cases, they should recommend that their client visit the doctor.

When estheticians recognize dermatitis, first she should ask the client about possible reasons for their current skin problem. Ask if she or he ate unusual food or started using a new skin care product that could cause the problem. If the reason was a chemical factor, such as cosmetic, cleaning product, detergent, etc., the client should be advised to immediately stop using it. In the case of a food allergy, a cleansing flush is recommended to remove the allergen from the body. The flushing method refers to drinking a large amount of water and colon cleansing with herbal supplements or a colonic procedure. Colonics may provide immediate relief due to efficient bowel cleansing action.

Light, calming facials can be very beneficial to relieve the mild symptoms of dermatitis. But you have to be aware, only a medical professional can treat severe cases of dermatitis.

The Calming Facial should include a light cleansing, herbal compress, light massage with healing moisturizer, and a calming mask.

Dermatitis Relief (Facial Procedure)

Before you consider doing a facial for a person with a dermatitis skin condition, you should know that no steaming or extraction should be allowed by any means. Use of hot towels and aromatherapy is strictly prohibited as well.

> Step #1: Clean the skin.

Start with Gentle Cleansing Gel (Raya Laboratories, Inc.) to clean the skin. Gentle Cleansing Gel is aloe-based and specially designed for dry and sensitive skin. Six herbal extracts are included in the cleansers that are known for their mild cleansing properties. It helps to moisturize, purify, and calm the skin. If the skin care line that you have been using has a good cleanser for sensitive skin you can use it for dermatitis treatment as well. Gently remove the cleanser with damp sponges or washcloths.

> Step #2: Use a mild astringent.

Follow with a mild herbal astringent or toner for sensitive skin. You can prepare your own toner using cosmetic and pharmaceutical ingredients.

Herbal Astringent Recipe
Boric acid (powder form) -1/4 teaspoon (5 g)
Distill water -2 oz (60 g)
Add 1 teaspoon (15 g) of glycerin

Add 1 ounce (30g) Calendula tincture (refer to the Chapter 5 for the method of preparation)
Mix it together in glass container and store it in cool and dry place.

This astringent has soothing and calming properties to relieve itchiness and irritation. The Boric acid acts as an antibacterial agent and can be purchased as an over-the-counter product at the local drugstore.

> Step #3: Follow with an herbal compress.

For this you need pre-cut gauze mask to saturate it in the herbal infusion. Or you can make the mask from gauze or cheesecloth. Herbal infusion is basically a tea. However, to steep the herb, you have to use boiling water.

Herbal Infusion Recipe
In small pot, combine 2 cups of water and 1 oz of dry Chamomile herb. Bring to boil.
Cover it and leave to steep for 10-15 min. (Or you can just add boiling water to the dry herb in the cup and steep it for 10 min.)
After the infusion has cooled off, saturate the gauze mask with the warm herbal infusion and apply on the client's face for 15 min.

I personally like to use Chamomile or Calendula herb, but other herbs, like sage or oak bark, also work very well. You can make infusions from two or three different herbs; it can only add benefits to the treatment.

Boric Acid Compress Recipe
Boric acid solution can be excellent calming compress if used it on its own. Take 1/2 tablespoon of Boric Acid and dissolve it into 2 ounces of distill water at room temperature. Saturate gauze mask with the solution and apply directly onto the face for 15 min.

> Step #4: Apply the calming mask.

The final step of dermatitis treatment is a calming mask application. Calming mask includes a Hydrocortisone 1% and Lanolin based cream.

Calming Mask Recipe
To make the mask, take one half of 1 oz. 1% Hydrocortisone ointment tube and mix it with 1 oz of Lanolin facial cream.

You can prepare Lanolin cream yourself at very easy steps. Lanolin cream is an excellent moisturizer that can be used to treat extremely dry skin and after microdermabrasion to heal redness and irritation quickly. It is a very simple formula that can be easily prepared at home or in the salon.

<u>Lanolin Moisturizer Recipe</u>
2 oz bee's wax
2 oz liquid lanolin
12 oz cacao butter
4 oz almond oil (substitute 2 oz of almond oil with 2 oz of jojoba oil for oily skin)
1 cup of distills water.

Combine bee wax, lanolin, and cacao butter in small pot and heat it on low heat (70-73 C) until they melt, while constantly stirring. Take it from the stove and slowly add oil while constantly stirring with mixer, and then slowly add water until the whole content becomes a harder consistency. If it's still too liquid, you can add more water; if it's too hard, you can add more oil. Let it cool off and check again if it is the correct consistency. Add water or oil to receive the desired results of a creamy lotion. You can add few drop of vitamin E oil, and few drops of essential oils, like sweet orange or jasmine for a pleasant smell. In fact, orange essential oil has anti-wrinkle properties, but do not put too much, since it can be irritating. Just a few drops are enough.

Here, there is no end to your creativity. I personally like to add jojoba oil or jojoba butter. It is excellent for dry and sensitive skin. You can also replace water with Aloe Vera gel and mix it with equal parts of distilled water. Use a blender or mixer to mix all ingredients. This formula can also serve as a massage cream for anti-aging lymph-drainage massages. For massage cream, you can make it a little more liquid, adding more oil like sunflower, olive oil, or wheat germ oil.

As an alternative to a mask with 1% Hydrocortisone ointment, you can prepare other calming masks with aloe vera gel.

<u>Using Aloe Vera</u>

The aloe vera plant contains the most miraculous ingredients of all time. Known for its potent leaves, aloe vera has been used as a medicinal herb for centuries. Some of important discoveries belong to Russian scientists who have found that aloe vera extract can regenerate nerve fibers. The pulp or gel contains 96% water and 4% "biological stimulator" that has healing and regenerating properties.

Fresh aloe vera gel is one of the best soothing and healing substances, and it appears to be a "must- have" ingredient for many cosmetic formulations. For the most benefits of this miracle plant, I recommend using pure aloe vera gel that you can obtain from your own aloe plant. Most commercial formulas contain preservatives that ruin the healing ingredients of aloe vera gel. Fresh pulp or gel can be used for soothing and nourishing treatments by adding them to masks or creams.

Aloe Vera Mask Recipe
For the dermatitis treatment, you can use fresh aloe vera gel (1 teaspoon), Calendula infusion, and 1/2 tube of Hydrocortisone cream. Mix all of the ingredients in the blender and use it as a soothing mask for dermatitis treatments.

> Step #5: Gently remove the mask.

To finish the treatment remove mask with damp cloth and gently massage face for 2 min with 1% Hydrocortisone ointment to make sure that it completely absorbed by skin.

Several sessions are recommended to relieve dermatitis. Up to five treatments every day or every other day are preferred. Advise your client use 2 % Hydrocortisone cream at home for faster improvement. If symptoms persist, refer your client to a medical professional for assistance.

Psoriasis

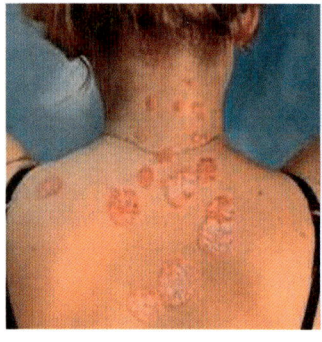
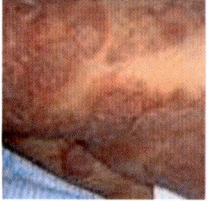

Psoriasis begins most often in people aged 10 to 40. However, people in all age groups are susceptible. Psoriasis is a chronic, recurring disease that causes one or more raised, red patches that have silvery scales and a distinct border between the patch and normal skin.

It usually starts as one or more small patches on the scalp, elbows, knees, back, or buttocks. The first patches may clear up after a few months or remain, sometimes growing together to form larger patches. Some people never have more than one or two small patches, and others have patches covering large areas of the body. Thick patches or patches on the palms of the hands, soles of the feet, or skin folds of the genitals are more likely to itch or hurt. However, many times a person has no symptoms. Although the patches do not cause extreme physical discomfort, they are very obvious and often embarrassing to the person. When psoriasis develops on the hands and feet, it is often difficult for people to perform daily tasks, such as picking up objects, typing, and walking. The itching and pain caused by psoriasis also makes daily life difficult.

The cause of psoriasis, which is an inflammatory skin condition, is not fully understood, but medical research has come to the conclusion that psoriasis starts with the immune system. Normally, the immune system defends the body from infection by bacteria, viruses, and other invaders. Sometimes, however, the immune system makes a mistake and attacks the cells, tissues, and organs of a person's own body. When this happens, the resulting disease is called an autoimmune disease.

Ask anyone with psoriasis what triggers a flare-up, and stress is likely to top the list. Scientific studies confirm that stress can worsen psoriasis and increase itching. Some people can even trace their first outbreak to a particularly stressful event.

Winter tends to be the most challenging season for people living with psoriasis. Numerous studies indicate cold weather is a common trigger for many people and that hot and sunny climates appear to clear the skin.

Psoriasis persists throughout life, but it may come and go. Symptoms are often diminished during the summer when the skin is exposed more to sunlight. One of the method therapy based on exposure to the ultraviolet light is phototherapy, and it can help clear up psoriasis for several months at a time.

Treatment for Psoriasis

Unfortunately, none of the available treatments for psoriasis are a cure. Treatment can often control the disease for long periods, but the disease can come back when treatment stops. In general, dermatologists treat psoriasis in three steps.

- Step #1: Medications applied to the skin (topical steroid medication, moisturizers with aloe vera, vitamin E and D, tar compounds)
- Step #2: Treatments that use light (photo therapy)
- Step #3: Medications given as a pill or injection (drugs related to vitamin A and D)

Psoriasis is very serious skin condition and has to be treated by skin care professional only.

Seborrheic Dermatitis

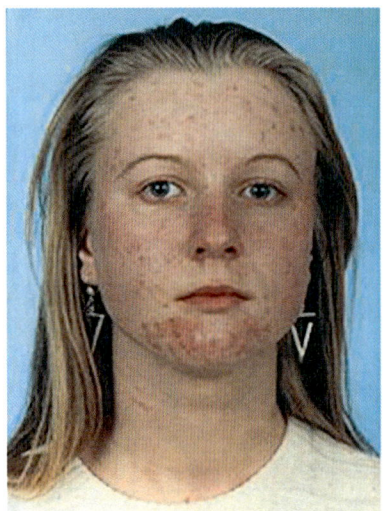
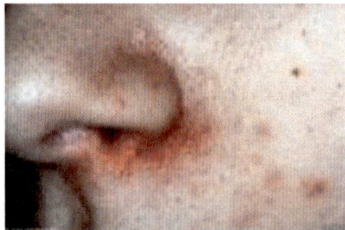

Scaly patches of skin that result from a disorder of sebaceous glands characterize *seborrhea or seborrheic dermatitis*. The initial symptoms begin with a significant oil production increase on the skin and hair. The pores getting clogged and comedones will form on the t-zone of the skin. The hair getting greasy too fast can create a large amount of dandruff. Seborrheic skin may be yellowish and greasy or dry and flaky. The skin disease usually starts at the puberty age and may last throughout adulthood. In adults, seborrheic dermatitis usually affects the scalp, eyebrows, ear canals, sides of the nose, and behind the ears. It sometimes affects the armpits, chest and in the groin area. Most people with the skin disorder complain of dandruff, especially on the back and sides of the scalp. Adult seborrhea is often associated with stress or mental disturbance. It also can be related to the hormonal imbalance, digestive system disorder, or/and a weak immune system. Other factors associated with an increased chance of developing seborrheic dermatitis include oily skin, obesity, acne, rosacea, and psoriasis.

The person's skin with seborrhea appears to be always greasy or dry with numerous of inflamed pustules and comedones located on the face, neck and the back. Very often you can see on the client with oily seborrhea big nodules that are fairly large (up to 1cm in diameter) and are inflamed. The treatment requires a therapeutical dose of antibiotics along with a nutritional program. Estheticians should be very careful to treat seborrhea. In severe cases, the best idea is to refer a client to the dermatologist for proper medical evaluation.

Skin Tags and Warts

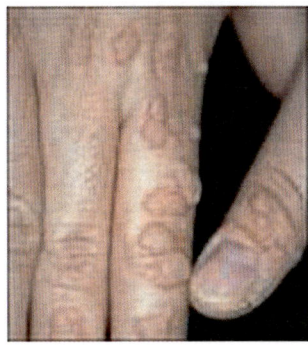
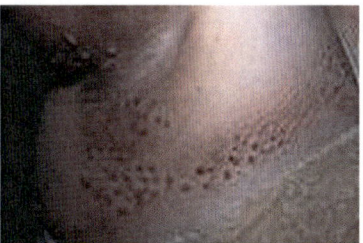

Skin Tags

A skin tag is a common, acquired benign skin growth that looks like a small piece of hanging skin. Skin tags are often described as bits of skin or flesh-colored tissue that project from the surrounding skin as a small, narrow stalk. They typically occur in locations including the neck, underarms, eyelids, and under the breasts. Although skin tags may vary somewhat in appearance, they are usually smooth or slightly wrinkled and irregular, flesh-colored or slightly brown and they hang from the skin on a small stalk. Sometimes skin tags may become fairly large in size and can become as big as a grape. Since skin tags are prevalent to arise more readily in areas of skin that have friction or rubbing, they are commonly seen in overweight people.

Treatment is usually not necessary unless the cutaneous tags are irritating or cosmetically displeasing. The growths may be removed with surgery by snipping with scissors, by freezing (cryotherapy), or by electrical burn (cautery or electrocoagulation). Electrocoagulation is the most common method of removing skin tags, and many skin tags removal devices operate from producing elect currents on the tip of the needle that can burn the skin. Skin tags do not have nerve endings, so the process is basically painless. But the spot can bleed slightly and require application of a disinfecting solution or bandage.

In some states, estheticians are allowed perform skin tags removing procedures. However, she or he has to complete a special course and learn how to use the equipment. Equipment is usually not very expensive and can be purchased directly from the manufacturer. Some manufacturers offer classes along with purchase.

Warts

Warts are a harmless skin growths caused by a type of virus called the human papillomavirus (HPV). There are more than 100 known types of HPV. HPV infects the top layer of skin, usually entering the body in an area of broken skin. The virus causes the top layer of skin to grow rapidly, forming a wart. Warts can grow anywhere on the body, and they are mostly common among children and young adults.

Warts are easily spread by direct contact with a human papillomavirus. The individual who has the virus can infect another person by sharing towels, razors, or other personal items. After contact with HPV, it can take 2 to 9 months of slow growth beneath the skin before someone notices a wart formation. Not every person can be infected by HPV virus though direct contact with the virus carrier. It directly depends on one's immune system strength and possibly other factors.

Warts come in a wide range of shapes and sizes. A wart may be a bump with a rough surface, or it may be flat and smooth. Tiny blood vessels grow into the core of the wart to supply it with blood. In both common and plantar warts, the blood vessels may look like dark dots in the wart's center. Warts are usually painless. But a wart that grows in a spot where you put pressure, such as on a finger or on the bottom of the foot, can be painful.

Types of Warts

All human warts can be classified into 5 types. They are:

> Type #1: Common Warts
> Common warts grow most often on the hands, but they may be anywhere on the body. They are rough, shaped like a dome, and gray-brown in color.

> Type #2: Plantar Warts
> Plantar warts grow on the soles of the feet. They look like hard, thick patches of skin with dark specks. Plantar warts may cause pain when you walk, and they may require possible surgical removal.

> Type #3: Flat Warts
> Flat warts usually grow on the face, arms, or legs. They are small and have flat tops with pink, light brown, or light yellow color.

> Type #4: Filiform Warts
> Filiform usually grow around the mouth, nose, or beard area. They are the same color as your skin and have growths that look like threads sticking out of them.

> Type #5: Periungual Warts
> Periungual warts grow under and around the toenails and fingernails. They look like rough bumps with an uneven surface and border.

Treatment of Warts

Most warts go away within months or years on their own and don't need treatment. But if person has warts that are painful or spreading, the treatment choices include:

- Using a home treatment such as salicylic acid or adhesive tape. One can get these without a prescription
- Putting a stronger medicine on the wart or getting a shot of medicine in it
- Freezing the wart (cryotherapy)
- Removing the wart with surgery (electro surgery, curettage, laser surgery)

Unfortunately, wart treatment does not always work. Even after a wart shrinks or goes away, warts may come back or spread to other parts of the body. This is because most treatments destroy the wart, but they do not kill the virus that causes the wart.

Molluscum Contagiosum

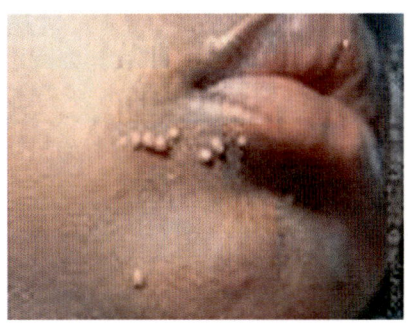
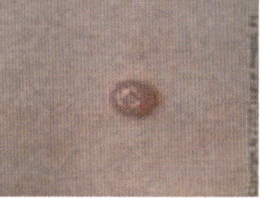

Molluscum contagiosum is contagious skin disease, and it can be contracted through nonsexual contact. This infection is transmitted through daily, intimate physical contact of any kind. For example, individuals who share towels have reported cases of molluscum contagiosum.

As a viral infection, molluscum contagiosum is caused by the existence of a harmful virus within the human body. Outbreaks are often noticeable on the abdomen, sexual genitalia, thighs, knees and buttocks. This skin infection is very easy recognizable because of the round and firm, flesh colored bumps that will be visible on any affected area of the body. These bumps, which may have a dimple in the center, are called papules. Many times, the papules will have a soft center that is filled with fluid.

Affected persons may also notice painful sores or skin lesions. If the patient scratches the bumps, or papule, it may evolve in linear formations and will spread to larger areas of the affected region. When molluscum contagiosum outbreaks have diminished, some patients will notice pit-like scars on the surface of the skin.

Children tend to get molluscum more often than adults. It is common in young children who have not yet developed immunity to the virus. Children also tend to have more direct skin-to-skin contact with others.

Treatment of Molluscum contagiosum

Treatment is not always necessary for children because molluscum contagiosum usually goes away on its own, without leaving a scar. Whether or not to treat depends on many factors. For example, if a bump is near a child's eye, it may be treated to prevent conjunctivitis or it may not be treated to avoid possible eye damage. Pain caused by treatment and the potential for scarring are important considerations when deciding about treatment for children.

Treatment for molluscum is similar to that for warts. Growths can be frozen with liquid nitrogen, destroyed with various acids or blistering solutions, or treated with an electric needle (electrocautery) and scraped off with a sharp instrument (curette). Laser therapy also has been effective in treating molluscum. All of these treatments can be performed in a dermatologist's office. If there are many growths, treatment sessions may be needed every 3 to 6 weeks until the growths disappear.

Ringworm

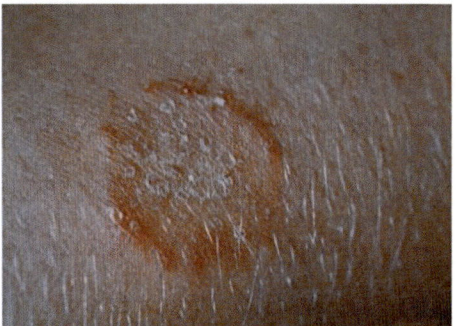

Ringworm (tinea) is a fungal skin infection caused by several different fungi and generally classified by its location on the body. Despite its name, ringworm infection does not involve worms. The name arose because of the ring-shaped skin patches created by the infection. Symptoms vary depending on the location of the infection. Dermatologists can frequently identify a ringworm infection by its appearance. Most often, there is little or no inflammation on the infected areas. An infected person may have itchy with a scaling, slightly raised border ring-shaped spot. These patches can come and go intermittently. The most commonly affected area of the body includes head, skin, and nails. Ringworm is contagious. It spreads when you have skin-to-skin contact with a person or animal that has it. It can also spread when you share things like towels, clothing, or sports gear.

Fortunately, Ringworm is an easy to treat skin problem and can clear up with oral and topical fungus-killing medicine. The medicine can be in taken in tablet or liquid form by mouth or as a cream applied directly to the affected area. If ringworm is not treated, skin may blister, and the cracks could become infected with bacteria.

If you, as an esthetician see some suspicious skin irritation, you can examine it using a Wood's lamp. Ringworm is usually seen under a Wood's lamp as a green, fluorescent, ring-looking patch. Refer your client to the dermatologist if you recognize such skin infection. Do not intend to treat the client's skin since infection can spread and cause further damage.

Keloid Scars

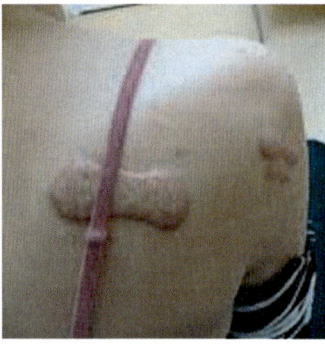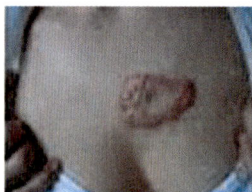

Keloids are raised overgrowths of scar tissue that occur at the site of a skin injury. They occur after trauma, surgical incisions, blisters, vaccinations, acne, chickenpox, or even minor scratches. Less commonly, keloids may form in places where the skin has not had a visible injury. Keloids differ from normal mature scars in composition and size. Some people are prone to keloid formation and may develop them in several places.

Keloid scars are shiny, smooth, and rounded skin elevations that may be pink, purple, or brown. They can be doughy, firm, or rubbery to the touch, and they often feel itchy, tender, or uncomfortable. Large keloids in the skin over a joint may interfere with joint function.

There is no single treatment for keloids, and most treatments do not give completely satisfying results. Two or more treatments may be combined. If you decide to pursue treatment for a keloid scar, you will have the best results if you start treatment soon after the keloid appears.

Keloid Scar Treatment

Available treatments include the following:

- Removal with Conventional Surgery

    This unreliable technique requires great care, and scars that return after being removed may be larger than the original. Keloids return in more than 45% of people when they are removed surgically. Keloids are less likely to return if surgical removal is combined with other treatments.

- Corticosteroid Injections

    Injections with triamcinolone acetonide or another corticosteroid medicine typically are repeated with intervals of four to six weeks.

This treatment can often reduce keloids size and irritation, but injections are uncomfortable.

- Cryotherapy

    This freezing treatment with liquid nitrogen is repeated every 20 to 30 days. It can cause a side effect of lightening the skin color, which limits this treatment's usefulness.

- Laser Therapy

    This is an alternative to conventional surgery for keloids removal. There is no good evidence that keloids are less likely to recur after laser therapy than after regular surgery.

Here I want to emphasize the importance of asking your client about predisposition to keloid before considering microdermabrasion treatment. Procedures like microdermabrasion cannot be performed on people with such skin disorders. So ask your client if they have keloid predisposition, and if they do not know, ask if any member of their family has it since it appears to have genetic roots. When keloids formation runs in a family, it usually affects several members. This can help you to make your decision on the skin treatment.

Acne Scarring

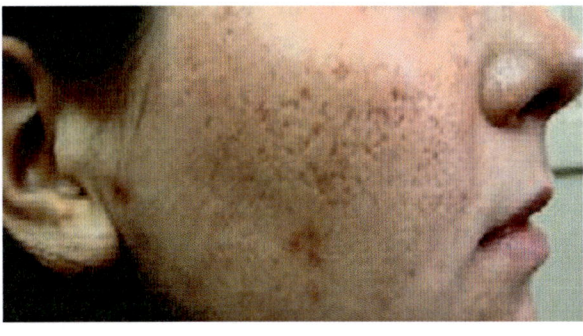
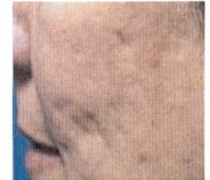

Scars (also called cicatrices) are areas of fibrous tissue that replace normal skin (or other tissue) after injury. A scar results from the biologic process of wound repair in the skin and other tissues of the body. Thus, scarring is a natural part of the healing process. With the exception of very minor lesions, every wound (e.g. after accident, disease, or surgery) results in some degree of scarring. There are two basic types of scars: older, "mature" scars that are pale or white in color, and newer scars, that still bear the red or purple tint from a recent trauma to the skin.

Acne is a skin condition that affects up to 80% of people in their teens and twenties and up to 5% of older adults. While many people recover from acne without any permanent effects, some people are left with disfiguring acne scars.

After an acne lesion has healed, it can leave a red or hyper-pigmented mark on the skin. This is actually not a scar, but rather a post-inflammatory change. The redness or hyper pigmentation is seen as the skin goes through its healing and remodeling process, which takes approximately 6-12 months. If no more acne lesions develop in that area, the skin can heal normally. Any color change or skin defect still present after 1 year is considered to be a permanent defect or scar.

There are some topical skin care products and medications that can improve mild scarring, but most acne scars are treated with a combination of some type of skin resurfacing. Severe scars can be removed by a surgical procedure called laser resurfacing. Mild acne scars can be successfully treated by microdermabrasion or a chemical peel, especially if scars are still new and fresh. For detailed treatment protocol, refer to **Chapter 8: "Microdermabrasion and Chemical Peels."**

Stretch Marks

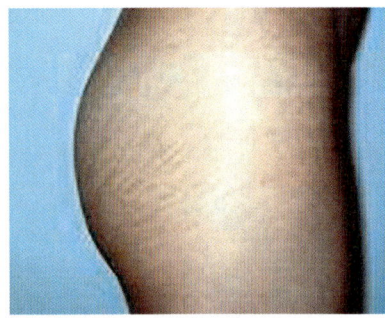
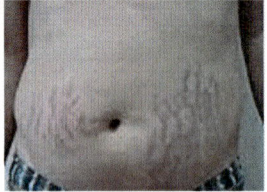

Stretch marks are a normal part of puberty for most girls and guys. When a person grows or gains weight rapidly (like during puberty), that person may get fine lines on the body called stretch marks. Stretch marks happen when the skin is pulled by rapid growth or stretching. Although the skin is usually fairly elastic, when it's overstretched, the normal production of collagen (the major protein that makes up the connective tissue in your skin) is disrupted. As a result, scars called stretch marks may form.

Stretch marks (striae) are pink, red, or purple indented streaks that often appear on the abdomen, breasts, upper arms, buttocks, and thighs. Depending on your skin color, the marks start out as pink, reddish brown, or dark brown streaks. The reddish-brown pigmentation in the marks gradually fades, and the stretch marks or "striae" begin to look like glistening silvery lines of scar tissue. Stretch marks are also very common in pregnant women, especially during the last half of pregnancy. People who are obese often have stretch marks. Bodybuilders are prone to getting stretch marks because of the rapid body changes that bodybuilding can produce.

The person can be concerned about these bright streaks on the skin, but stretch marks are not serious and fade over time. In some cases, however, widespread stretch marks are a sign of a medical condition such as Cushing's syndrome or other adrenal gland disease.

There are some effective methods to treat or at least diminish stretch marks on the skin. Stretch marks creams can lessen the appearance of stretch marks, but won't completely remove them. The microdermabrasion procedure however, can significantly reduce stretch marks and will promote smoother skin. The effect of the procedure can be seen and felt right away. Most microdermabrasion procedures take more than one session. This would depend on the rigorousness of the scars on the skin.

Cellulite

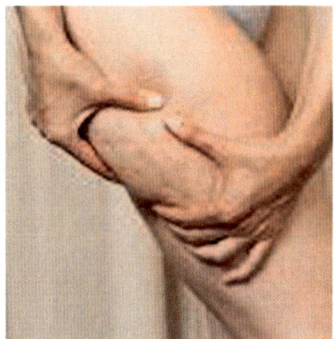

Cellulite is the lumpy substance resembling cottage cheese that is commonly found on the thighs, stomach, and buttock. The lumpiness of cellulite is caused by fat deposits that push and distort the connective tissues beneath the skin, leading to the characteristic changes in appearance of the skin.

Underneath the dermis and epidermis are three specific layers of fat. Cellulite tends to develop in the subcutaneous fat layers. This layer of fat is unique in its structure compared to the other layers because its fatty parts are structured into specific chambers by strands of linked tissue around it.

Cellulite is much more common in women than in men because of the differences in the way fat, muscle, and connective tissue are distributed in the skin of men versus women. Most people dislike the appearance of cellulite and prefer to have skin as smooth as they possibly can.

Regular exercise and well balanced diets do not always reverse or prevent its formation, although an unhealthy lifestyle will make the overall appearance worse over time, due to poor nutrition, weight gain, and lack of sufficient water intake.

There are many anti-cellulite creams available on the market that contain herbs, antioxidants, minerals, and vitamins. These assist the skin to become softer, healthier, and smoother and allow it to repair itself more easily. Creams that contain herbs like green tea, guarana and cayenne pepper are more effective when treating cellulite, as they increase skin's blood circulation. Creams containing anti-inflammatory agents can also assist with improving lumpy-looking skin.

The areas that are affected by cellulite are usually dry and damaged; therefore they need additional moisture to improve skin condition. Increasing moisture in the affected area since the affected skin may appear too dry and damaged can temporarily reduce the appearance of cellulite.

There are many cellulite-reducing types of equipment that have been advertised and promoted by cosmetic companies. The cellulite treatment machines are based either on mechanical massage, micro current, radio frequency or infrared light therapy. Microdermabrasion treatment has been also claimed to help with the cellulite problems, but from my experience, microdermabrasion procedures do not provide long-term effects.

The most effective anti-cellulite machines are the ones that use infrared light and/or radio frequency waves. Infrared energy is a heat, and the radio frequency (RF) energies work together to drive the heat deeper, loosening the connections between fat pockets and also stimulating collagen production.

The cellulite treatment procedure is an excellent addition to any esthetic business. However, before investing in expensive equipment, do your own research as to which product/equipment has the most positive reviews. Visit an annual esthetician show (Las Vegas, Long Beach, and etc.) where you can experience the equipment by yourself and talk to other people who are already working with some. Visiting annual esthetic conferences are the most effective way to stay on top of newest technology in skin care industry. I highly recommend all skin care professionals to attend an esthetic conference at least once per year.

If you notice, I did not describe any of the most important skin problems that esthetician deal with on regular basis; Acne vulgaris, Hyperpigmentation, Rosacea, and Skin Aging. Those require more attention and detailed studies. I decided to dedicate separate chapters for each of those more common skin problems.

Chapter 4: Acne Vulgaris

Acne Vulgaris (commonly called acne) is the common skin condition that is caused by inflammation of sebaceous glands. Acne primarily develops from blocked pilosebaceous canals. The sebaceous canals get plagued by hardened sebum (skin oil), and dead cells, therefore, provide a breeding environment for staphylococcus and propionibacterium acne bacteria. The surrounding area gets inflamed and irritated. Inflammation near the skin's surface produces a pustule; deeper inflammation results in a papule; and the deeper still it becomes a cyst. Blackheads are the result of an oil oxidizing process that causes the oil color to change.

Acne is closely related to seborrhea, which appears to be one of the important factors of acne development. In fact, the most common and severe form of seborrhea is acne vulgaris. It is the chronic inflammation of sebaceous glands and hair follicles, caused by staphylococcus bacteria.

Another reason for acne is a tiny parasite found in sebaceous glands and hair follicles called *demodex folliculorum*. This very small parasite is present in almost all skin types, but the most common it is shown in is oily skin. Development of acne depends on the individual tolerance to the parasite and acne bacteria (propiobacterium). People with strong immune systems and that are generally healthy are unlikely will to have acne skin disease. In contrary, people suffering from chronic intestinal, liver, and stomach diseases are more susceptible to the bacteria that cause acne. Lastly, research shows that acne can also have a genetic predisposition for some individuals whose family members also suffered from this skin disorder.

Acne vulgaris is characterized by the appearance of comedones, papules, pustules, and nodules in more severe acne form. A comedone is a whitehead (closed comedone) or a blackhead (open comedone) without any clinical signs of inflammation. Papules and pustules are raised bumps with obvious inflammation.

The face and upper neck are the most commonly affected areas, but the chest, back, and shoulders may have acne as well. Some of the large nodules sometimes called "cysts" and the term nodulocystic have been used to describe severe cases of inflammatory acne. It mostly happens when oil glands come to life around puberty, stimulated by male hormones from the adrenal glands of both boys and girls.

Four Stages of Acne

There are four stages of acne that you as a skin care professional have to be familiar with:

> Stage #1: Comedonal Acne
> In comedonal acne, no inflammatory lesions are present. Comedonal lesions ("blackheads") are the earliest sign of acne, and they are the precursor of inflammatory lesions.

> Stage #2: Mild Inflammatory Acne
> Mild inflammatory acne is characterized by the presenting of inflammatory papules and comedones.

> Stage #3: Moderate Inflammatory Acne
> Moderate inflammatory acne condition contains comedones, inflammatory papules, and pustules.

> Stage #4: Nodulocystic Acne
> Comedones, inflammatory lesions, and large nodules greater than 5 mm in diameter characterize Nodulocystic acne. Scarring is often evident.

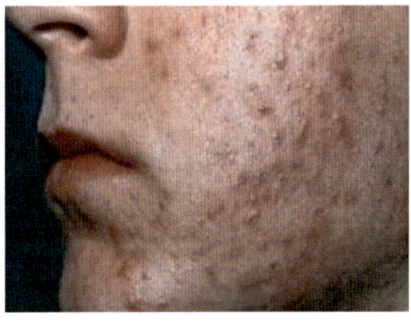
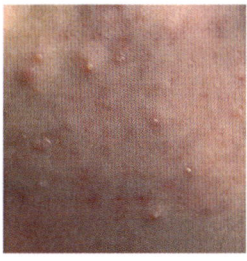

Acne can affect all age groups, from a few months after birth to the elderly. During puberty, virtually all boys and 90% of girls will have some spots and pimples, which are usually mild forms of acne. A hormonal changes in teenage boys, characterized by excessive testosterone production, contributes to abnormal function of oil glands. High levels of the male hormone, testosterone, excites the oil sebaceous glands (oil glands) to produce more amount of oily substance sebum.

Adult acne is becoming more and more common, so common, in fact that 25% of adult men and 50% of adult women are affected by it. Appearance of acne in adults has the same root as teenage acne: hormonal imbalance. Some adult women experience mild to moderate acne due to hormonal changes associated with pregnancy, menstruation, and stopping or starting birth control pills. That is why women suffering from adult acne notice a change in their skin around the time of their menstrual cycle. It is known those two weeks before menstruation, woman's estrogen levels decrease while progesterone levels begin to rise. This causes the sebaceous glands to produce more oil, which can result in the onset of pimples.

Symptoms of hormone imbalance are caused primarily by the incorrect relationship between progesterone and estrogen levels in the body. The two female hormones, estrogen and progesterone, exist in a delicate balance. Variations in that balance can have a dramatic effect on your health, resulting in symptoms of hormone imbalance. The amounts of these hormones that the woman's body produces from month to month may vary, depending on factors, such as stress, nutrition, exercise, and most importantly, lack of ovulation, caused by taking birth control pills. In addition, women often have stressful lives, eat processed foods, or skip meals. Some may take synthetic estrogen HRT (hormone replacement therapy) or have had hysterectomies. All these factors can add more estrogen to the female body, resulting in excess estrogen, which will cause hormone imbalance symptoms.

Thousand of product and varieties of acne treatment have been offered by allopathic and holistic medicine. Unfortunately, esthetic acne treatments come too late for people with acne skin disorder. Most acne sufferers rush to see dermatologist to get a prescription drug. I believe it happens due to the fact that domestic beauticians did not gain the reputation of being sufficiently educated in regards to acne treatments. Antibiotics that are prescribed by a dermatologist can help the problem for some time, but bacteria has tendency to accommodate to the medicine and develop immunity to the particular type of antibiotic. Besides, prolonged intake of antibiotics destroys immune systems that lead to further health problems.

In contrary, in European countries, acne sufferers first look for help not in doctor's office but from a cosmetologist-beautician. There are varieties of very effective esthetic acne treatments that provide excellent results to treat moderate to severe acne conditions. And I am going to reveal several protocols of the acne treatments further in this chapter.

Esthetic Acne Treatments

Proper diagnosis of acne skin problems is one of the most important tasks for skin care professionals. The most common, acne vulgaris, we are going to discuss with its first, second, and third stage. Patients with nodulocystic acne usually do not come to esthetician; they look for professional help from dermatologists. In my extensive practice, I have been able to deal with all types of acne, including nodulocystic acne. I am going to describe all of my acne facial protocols that show excellent results for treating this skin problem. However, let me say, it is definitely your choice whether or not try to use it in your practice or just to simply refer your clients with acne to the doctor's office.

From my 25 years of experience, I can certainly say that acne is the most responsive skin problem, which is something that I cannot say about hyperpigmentation or aging skin treatments. If you are going to use my techniques, your client will be able to see results after the first treatment.

Let start with the first stage of acne, which is characterized by localization of blackheads on the T-zone and chin. Some inflamed papules might be present as well. This condition can be mostly seen on teenagers in their puberty stage. But some adults may also develop comedones, due to hormonal imbalance or bad cosmetic product usage.

The initial consultation with a person who has acne is very important, since you have to be aware of all the reasons of acne development. Spend some time to observe the skin and talk about a person's lifestyle. Are there any previous attempts to treat acne? And what were the results? While observing the skin, you can ask several questions about eating habits, possible acne heredity, usage of skin care products at home, length of existing problem, main complaints, and so on. Recommending professional skin care products for home use is one of the important steps during consultation since a majority of acne sufferers are not aware of proper skin care regimen. It is essential that you carry cosmetic products for oily and problem skin types. To my knowledge, almost all professional skin care lines include some product for acne conditions. If you are looking for one, I can suggest you try excellent formulas from Raya Lab, Inc., such as Camphor Cleanser, Blemish Control Lotion, Bio-Drying Lotion, Bio-Drying Mask, and Vitamin B Moisturizer are effective antibacterial products that give immediate acne relief. Further in this chapter, I will give a few acne treatment formulas that you can prepare yourself, using pharmaceutical and herbal substances.

Here are important things that the client has to know about acne:

- Oil-based cosmetics and sunscreens may make acne worse.
- Squeezing pimples may damage the skin and cause scarring. Only skin care professionals can do proper extraction of comedones and blemishes. Healthy diet habit will contribute to acne's clear up.
- Acne skin care has to include Cleanser, Astringent, moisturizer for oily skin and Anti-bacterial mask.
- Hot water may aggravate acne due to excessive oil production
- Dedicated series of acne treatments is necessarily to see obvious results. Some students or people with low income cannot afford expensive facial treatments; I usually offer discounted prices for these treatments especially if they decide go for series of facials.

Protocol for Acne Treatment

➢ <u>Step #1: Cleanse.</u>

Apply Camphor Soufflé Cleanser or any another appropriate cleanser. Keep it on the client's face for 1-2 min massaging gently.

If you are using hot towels for your facials, it is not recommended to use it on acne that has acute inflammation signs, such the presence of pussy pustules and cysts.

Exfoliation with any scrubs or brushing is strongly prohibited for inflammation acne. But it is absolutely safe to use it for mild and moderate acne skin conditions.

➢ <u>Step #2: Exfoliate.</u>

Follow with gentle exfoliation with appropriate skin scrub. I personally like to use Bamboo Scrub (Raya Lab, Inc.). This herb-based exfoliating cream combines finely ground bamboo with jojoba beads and micro-fine French talc. It effectively removes dead cells of the epidermis and lifts away dull, dry skin to improve texture and healthy clarity. But, remember, for acne conditions with obvious inflammation (pussy and red pustules) exfoliation should be avoided.

➢ <u>Step #3: Extract.</u>

Gently remove the cleanser and turn on the steamer, while preparing the extraction mask.

Extraction Mask Recipe

I use a mixture of Camphor Soufflé, sea salt, and Hydrogen peroxide 3%. Dilute one part of camphor cleanser with one part of hydrogen peroxide and add a quarter of a teaspoon of sea salt.

Apply thin layer of the extraction mask and slightly massage it for 30 seconds around the acne locations. Leave it on while steaming the face. Steaming should last about 5-10 min. Remove the mask with cotton pads, saturated in Hydrogen peroxide solution.

Here I have to say few words about Hydrogen peroxide solution (3% H2O2). H2O2 is the chemical formula of the Hydrogen Peroxide. I use this product all the time; for extractions, for preparing facial masks, for disinfecting instrument, etc. In addition to its ability to cleanse wounds, peroxide is probably the best remedy to dissolve earwax. The same action it does for the comedones since comedones are oxidized oil. This inexpensive, over-the-counter solution has amazing properties for softening comedones by applying it to the skin directly. Plus, it has a strong oxidizing agent that has excellent antibacterial properties. Besides, 3% H2O2 provides cells with oxygen molecule to help with their regenerative abilities.

For the extraction you need a comedone extractor, needles, disposable cotton, gauze tissue, and 3% H202 solution. I use an extractor for especially hard to reach places, like the nose folds, chin, inside the ear, and between the eyebrows. But I prefer manual extraction with the index fingers wrapped in sterile gauze. If you are going to use the extraction mask along with steaming, skin pores will open well enough that hard squeezing is not necessary. Hard squeezing traumatizes skin and can leave marks or scars. Instead of squeezing, rather push fingers toward each other. Try to remove as many possible blackheads and whiteheads, while, from time to time, wiping the area with a saturated 3% H202 cotton ball.

If blood appears when you remove the pustule, immediately put the disinfectant solution (Calendula tincture) on the spot and keep until it stops bleeding. You can use 3% H202 as well.

After you are done with extraction, saturate a clean cotton ball with Calendula Lotion and wipe the entire face. Calendula flowers have amazing anti-inflammatory and healing properties. It contains provitamin A, vitamin D, oleanolic acid, and many other biologically important substances. Conditions on which to use calendula tincture or ointment can be quiet a broad: slow healing wounds, burns, sunburns, eczemas, tears, cuts, abrasions, chapped or chafed skin, inflamed mucous membranes, and skin inflamed lesions are just to name a few. Calendula extract stimulates the formation of new tissue, and its anti-inflammatory properties provide soothing effects, while gently promoting blood circulation.

My education makes me emotionally attached to natural pharmaceuticals substances rather than synthetic substances. Almost all of my formulas are based on herbal and over-the-counter pharmaceutical products combined. For many years, I have been searching for formulas that really work and give consistent effects, and I am willing to share with you how easy these formulas are to make your own professional products that really work.

Calendula Tincture Recipe and method of preparation

40% food grain alcohol (vodka) - 400mg

Dry Calendula flowers- 1 oz.

Add all together in glass container and keep in cool place for week before using it.

A tincture is an alcoholic extraction of herb. Alcohol extracts the active constituents out of the plant matter and acts as a preservative, allowing the tincture to retain its effectiveness for up to 2 years. Any part of the plant may be used. Place 4 ounces of dried herbs in a glass jar with a tight-fitting lid and add 2 cups of vodka (80proof food grain alcohol). Store it for two weeks in a cool place, shaking it occasionally. Strain the mixture using cheesecloth, and poor it into a brown glass bottle. It is ready to use.

Using method describing above you can prepare calendula tincture from dry calendula flowers available at any health food store. It usually sells in the bulk. One ounce of dry calendula flower will cost around three dollars. Then you have to purchase inexpensive vodka from your local liquor store. Vodka is 40% grain alcohol that I strongly prefer over rubbing alcohol.

Take 400mg of vodka (approximately two cups) and one ounce of dry calendula flowers. Keep mixture in glass jar or bottle and store it in cool place. Let it sit for 7-10 days. After that, the tincture is ready to use. Strain the mixture using cheesecloth and place the calendula lotion in any glass bottle.

I use calendula tincture in many of my facials. It is excellent disinfectant and healing solution. I use it for preparing anti-acne astringent and anti-inflammatory masks as well.

> Step #5: Healing Massage
> In my book, I am going to describe several types of facial massage techniques, including lymph-drainage facial massages for anti- aging treatments, plastic anti-aging massages, and healing massages.

Healing Massage

Healing massage is usually performed after extraction for acne treatments. The healing massage is recommended for oily and problem skin for the purpose of closing pores after extraction; to reduce sebum production and to diminish post-acne blemishes. You can use this type of massage only for mild to moderate acne conditions. But in case of severe skin inflammation and cystic acne, any massage is prohibited.

The technique requires you to use medicated powder (available at local pharmacy store) or unscented baby powder. You can also prepare massage powder according to the formula below:

Massage Powder Recipe

Cornstarch - 1 cup (240ml)
Baby powder - 2 tablespoons (1 oz)
Zinc oxide - 1 oz (30 g)
Alum powder - 1 teaspoon (5 g)

To begin massage take a small amount of medicated powder on your hands and spread it all over client's face. Begin with gliding stroke (effleurage) following skin lines according diagram below.

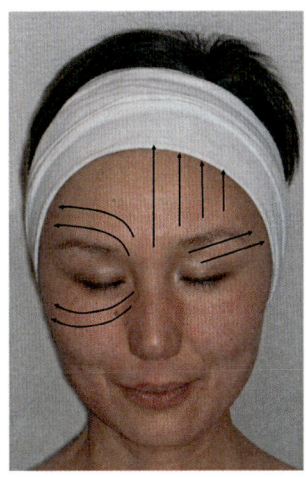
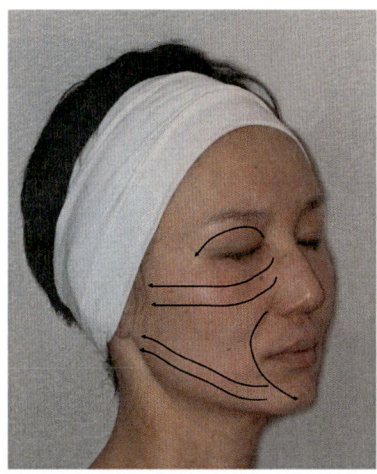

➢ Step #1: Effleurage.

This is a gliding stroke, performed with the four fingers of both hands kept together. Effleurage each skin line, starting from the forehead and heading down to the base of the neck. Repeat 3 times.

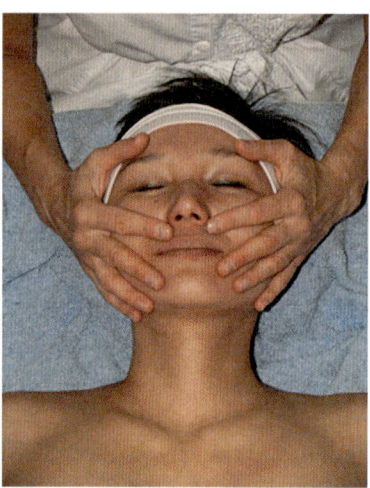

➢ Step #2: Petrissage.

This is a kneading motion, performed with index and thumb fingers. Slightly pinch folds of the skin between index finger and thumb, following the skin lines. Always start with the forehead.

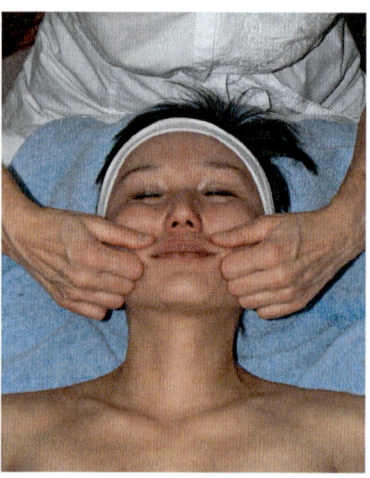

➢ Step #3: Kneading the nose muscles.

This is performed with thumbs of both hands keeping remained fingers under the chin. Duration is about 30 seconds.

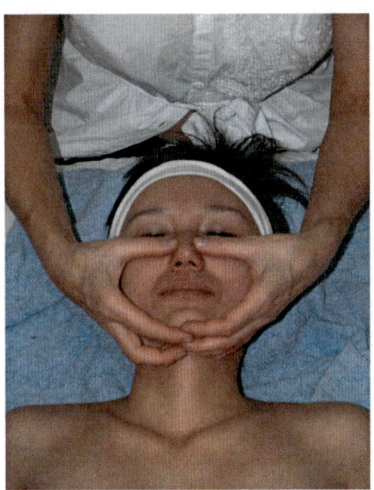

➢ Step #4: Kneading the forehead muscles.

This starts with the eyebrows heading upward to hairline, while slightly pinching skin between index fingers and thumbs. Repeat three times beginning from beginning of eyebrows up to hairline, than from middle part of eyebrows and from the end of eyebrows.

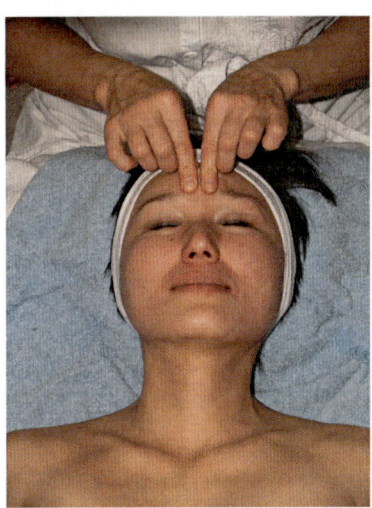

➤ Step #5: Vibration.

This is a kneading motion performing by pinching folds of the skin between thumb and knuckle of index finger adding light vibration to it. Follow the skin lines and repeat twice for entire face.

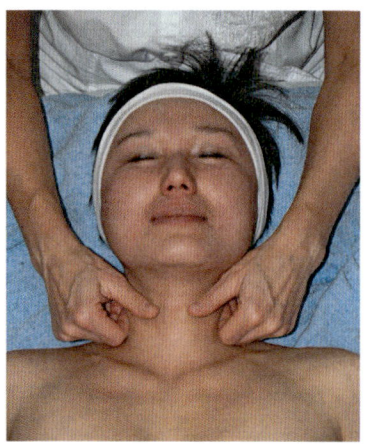 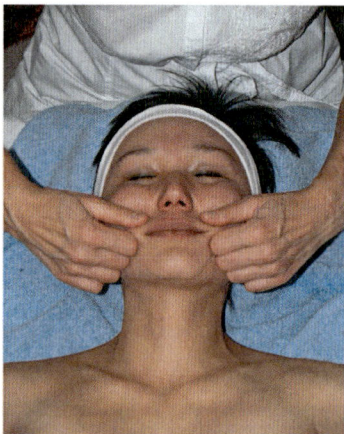

➤ Step #6: Percussion.

This is a light percussive motion all over the face by tips of all fingers of both hands.

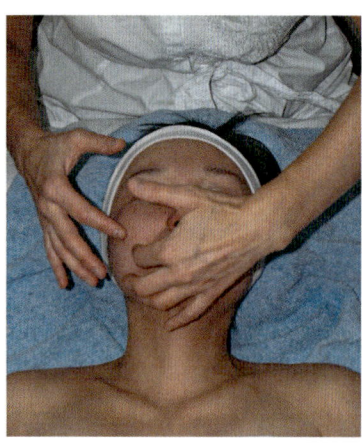 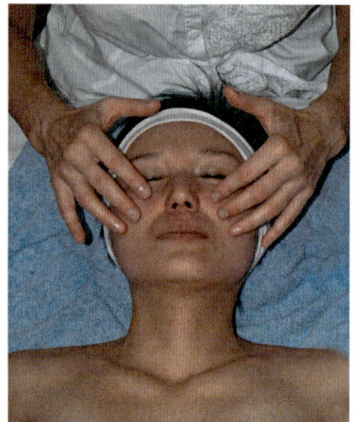

➤ Step #7: Effleurage.

Finish the massage with a light fingertip flutter and effleurage for entire face according skin lines.

The total duration of healing massage approximately 10 min.

For cases of mild to moderate acne, I usually follow up with a high frequency procedure. This is a very popular treatment, which may be applied directly or indirectly to the skin to stimulate healing processes. The high frequency electrical current enhances blood circulation, infuses skin with oxygen rich ozone molecules, and therefore kills bacteria that cause acne. Duration is 3-5 minutes. If there is any noble (a palpable solid lesion of the skin), apply direct current for 60-120 seconds for better results.

> Step #8: Apply an anti-acne mask.

Masks are the most effective cosmetic procedure that provides strong effects for the skin condition. It is moisturizing, nourishing, antibacterial cleansing, and calming that improves skin tremendously. Anti-acne masks should have antibacterial and healing properties in the first place. Also they work close to pores after extraction and improve skin color. I have designed a few formulations that I have been using with great success for years.

Duration of application is around 15-20 min.

Antibacterial Clay Mask Recipe

Purchase kaolin clay- facial mask in your local health food store. The nutritional company "Now" manufactures the product called "Kaolin Clay", and it comes in 4 oz jar. You can also purchase it online from many different vitamin companies. Kaolin Clay is a white powder, and it is absolutely a safe and natural substance. It has an excellent tightening and cleansing effect when used as a facial mask.

To make the anti-acne cleansing and disinfecting mask, measure one teaspoon of Kaolin and one tablespoon of 3% H_2O_2. For severe acne cases, you can dilute Kaolin with the Calendula Tincture that I have mentioned above. Just mix equal parts of each product.

I also like to add a 1/4-teaspoon of Boric acid powder that you can buy over-the-counter in your local drugstore. Boric acid works as a disinfectant and skin-calming agent.

Another ingredient that has superior tightening and antibacterial properties is alum powder or alum crystals. It is a tightening agent that can be added to the masks or astringents. Alum visibly diminishes larger pores and has excellent antibacterial properties.

You can purchase it either in powder or crystal form at health food stores or online.

Dilute crystals in hot water to make an alum solution. The Alum solution is a great base for the Kaolin mask, and it can be used for oily skin with enlarged pores. Indeed, alum is the only one pharmaceutical product that creates this amazing and highly desirable effect. Alum powder can be added to the clay mask to make tightening mask.

<u>*Alum Solution Recipe*</u>

Alum crystals -1 teaspoon (5 g)

Hot distill water or boiling tap water - 7 oz (200ml)

When you mix ingredients for clay mask make sure that the mask is not too runny and not too thick. It should be "sour cream"-like in consistency.

Apply the mask for 15-20 min or just simply leave it on until it dries. Do not wash the client's face with sponges and a bowl of water. Just use damp washcloths that I usually keep in my hot cabin. Cool off it before using for removing the mask.

If you feel like you do not want to mess with mask preparation, I can highly recommend that you use Bio-Drying Mask from Raya Lab, Inc. It is an excellent product that contains kaolin, aloe vera, and zinc oxide as its main ingredients. There are other great masks, called Bio-Sulfur Masque and Blemish Control Masque, which can be used in moderate and cystic stages of acne vulgaris.

There are several additional effective formulations that can be used for specific acne conditions. Some of them are the following:

<u>*White Clay Mask for mild Acne*</u>
Kaolin clay - one teaspoon (5 g)
Hydrogen peroxide 3% or Calendula lotion - 1 table spoon (15 g)
Boric acid powder - 1/4-teaspoon
Mix all together and apply on the face for 15-20 min

<u>*Clay Mask for Oily Skin*</u>
Kaolin clay - 1 teaspoon (5 g)
Hydrogen peroxide 3% or Calendula lotion - 1 tablespoon (15 g)
Add ¼ - teaspoon alum powder
Mix together and keep on the face for 15-20 min

Clay Mask with Ichtiolum for Cystic Acne

One tube of ichtiolum ointment 2% (over-the-counter at the pharmacy or drugstore)

Take 1/4 of the ichtiolum ointment 2% and add 1/4 teaspoon H202. Thoroughly mix it together and apply on the red, inflamed blemish for 20 min. It helps to reduce inflammation. This mix does have some strong smell, but it is very safe and effective product.

Mask for Oily Comedonic Skin

Kaolin clay –1 teaspoon (5 g)
Zinc oxide-1 teaspoon (5 g)
Boric acid powder ¼ of teaspoon
Alum solution for mixture
Add dry ingredient together and store in a separate container. For one treatment, use one teaspoon of mixture and add Alum solution for creamy consistency.

Blemish Control Mask with Sulfur

Kaolin - 2 oz (60 g)
Cornstarch - 1 teaspoon (5g)
Alum powder - 1/4 teaspoon
Boric acid powder - 1/4 teaspoon
Sulfur — 1/4 teaspoon
Mix all ingredients together and store in dry container. For one treatment, use one teaspoon of mixture and Calendula lotion to reach creamy consistency.

Seaweed (Spongilla) Mask

Spongilla powder - 1 teaspoon (5 g)
3% H202 - 1 tablespoon (15g)

Astringent for Enlarged Pores

You can use this lotion for mixing with Kaolin Clay to create a mask for oily comedone skin.

Alum powder - 1/4 teaspoon
Glycerin -1 teaspoon (15 g)
96% food grain alcohol (" Everclear" or 190 proof food grain alcohol) - 1 oz. (30ml)
Distilled water – 2 oz. (60 ml)
Add all ingredients and mix it very well. Store in glass container in a cool and dark place.

Mask with Egg Whites for Enlarged Pores
Bitted eggs white - one
Alum powder - ¼ teaspoon (1, 5 g)
Kaolin - 1 teaspoon (5 g)
Peppermint oil – few drops
Keep it on the face until it dries. Remove with lukewarm water.

Citric acid is a common ingredient in skin masks and some lotions. This ingredient is naturally found in citrus fruits. It easily mixes into liquids, making it a valuable cosmetic ingredient. Citric acid does have skin bleaching effects, and it can be added to any facial lotion or mask. You can purchase it at the grocery store or online: **www.NationalChemicals.com**

Bleaching Mask with Citric Acid
Kaolin clay 2 oz (50 g)
Citric acid crystals - 1/4 teaspoon
Camphor crystals – 1/2 teaspoon
Hydrogen peroxide 3% 1oz
Mix dry ingredients and store in dry container. Use one teaspoon of powder with 1 oz of 3% H_2O_2 to prepare the mask. The mask has great cleansing and bleaching properties. Do not use this mask for sensitive skin, because major irritation may occur.

Since this mask has the ability to double in size, store it in the big glass containers immediately after preparation and store the rest.

Drying and Disinfecting Mask
Kaolin Clay - 1 teaspoon (5g)
Zinc Oxide - 1 teaspoon (5g)
Glycerin - 1 teaspoon (5g)
Mix all ingredients and use immediately after preparation. The rest you can store and reuse later.

Mask with Allantoin - Calming Mask
Kaolin clay 1 oz
Allantoin powder 1/2 oz
Mix all dry ingredients with 1 oz of 3% H_2O_2.
Apply it for 15-20 min.

Mask for Extraction
Flax seeds meal – 1 teaspoon (5 g)
Kaolin - 1 teaspoon (5 g)
Hydrogen peroxide 3% – approximately 1 ounce

> Step #8: Finish Facial treatment with anti- bacterial moisturizer.

After mask is removed, apply oil-free moisturizer. Every good moisturizer and treatment product has the ultimate goal of regulating and stabilizing the skin's own acid mantle, a very thin layer of emulsified oil-and- water with slightly acidic PH. This mantle, or hydro-lipid film, varies according to skin condition and type. When a person has an acne condition, their skin has a strong acidic PH, and acne products have to be alkaline to restore proper PH. For acne treatment, I recommend alkaline, water-based moisturizer that carry antibacterial properties. Vitamin B Cream, designed by Raya Lab, Inc., is a highly effective moisturizer for oily and blemished skin. A mixture of natural botanical extracts, vitamins, and amino acids help to moisturize and balance the skin, while natural Vitamin B complex (Yeast Extract) helps to regulate oil gland secretion to reduce clogged pores and inflammations.

In severe cases of blemishes, I recommend that you do not use any moisturizer at all. On the contrary, put a small amount of medicated powder on the entire face. This way, it will keep down bacteria growth for several hours. It is very important to advise your client not to wash their face until the next morning to keep pores closed and allow the treatment to maximize its anti-inflammatory effect.

One treatment per week is usually recommended, even though improvement has been seen after the first treatment. Depending on acne condition, up to 20 treatments is advised to clear up the complexion.

Microdermabrasion to treat Acne Vulgaris

Microdermabrasion is a very effective treatment for reducing and controlling acne. However, as with other acne treatments, results differ between individuals. This is because causes and types of acne vary between people. Many people who have used microdermabrasion to treat acne have found that it works almost from the first day of use. Some users haven't found microdermabrasion to be very helpful at all in treating acne.

However, in most cases, microdermabrasion will reduce the appearance of acne scars; it improves the look of large pores, blackheads, whiteheads, acne, scars, brown marks, stretch marks, uneven tones, and fine wrinkles.

There are several different techniques used today, including varieties of microdermabrasion-style creams. Some traditional estheticians or treatment facilitators may still use high-pressure handheld machines to spray aluminum/zinc oxide crystals at the affected skin ("sandblasting") to exfoliate the skin. However, salons and clinics are increasingly turning to the "diamond peel" method. Diamond microdermabrasion is similar to the crystal method mentioned above with the dead skin and dirt sucked out through a vacuum tube but with a diamond-tipped rod or wand, used to polish the skin and remove the scar tissue, replacing the high-pressure crystal flow. This makes the diamond technique far more accurate and less irritating to the skin.

Treatment of acne with the diamond crystal-free system is a promising alternative to acne treatment facials. There is a strong indication that clients should be treated with the microdermabrasion procedure when they have acne scars. The contra-indication for this procedure is nobulecystic acne; the microdermabrasion is prohibited when skin is covered with pussy, red lesions and inflamed papules. Microdermabrasion is also not a good choice for those individuals with the following conditions: rosacea, herpes, warts, eczema, lupus, and diabetes. Microdermabrasion, on the other hand, gives excellent results for oily skin and, as I mentioned, skin with post acne scars and blemishes. It promotes new cells production in the deepest layer of the skin as it clears dull and congested skin.

I designed my Protocol for Microdermabrasion Acne treatment along with extraction before the actual microdermabrasion. It works more effective than doing extraction after microdermabrasion.

Protocol for Microdermabrasion Acne Treatment

> Step #1: Cleanse.

This is with Cleanser designed for problem and oily skin. If you like to use hot towels, you can follow with a hot towel application to soften comedones and open the pores. Scrub or exfoliation is not recommended, due to the risk of spreading bacteria on other skin parts.

> Step #2: Steam.

Steam face for 10 min following with 3%H_2O_2 application for whole face. Perform extraction with extractor or manually. Follow with Calendula Lotion to disinfect the skin. Apply few times all over the face, particularly on the affected area.

> Step #3: Extract.

Refer to the extraction technique at the acne treatment protocol.

> Step #4: Apply the microdermabrasion solution.

Microdermabrasion solution is needed to prepare skin for microdermabrasion in order to degrease the skin to achieve a deeper abrasive effect. I designed my own formula for microdermabrasion solution that contains a few pharmaceutical ingredients that you can easy find in the pharmacy or drugstore.

> *Microdermabrasion Skin Preparation Solution Recipe*
>
> *To prepare 8oz of the microdermabrasion solution, you need:*
>
> *3 oz (100ml) 96% grain alcohol ("Everclear" (190 proof food grain alcohol) is available at any liquor store.)*
>
> *Calendula Tincture - 3 oz (100ml)*
>
> *Salicylic acid powder - 1 teaspoon (5g)*
>
> *2 oz of Camphor Spirits (two small bottles).*
>
> *Mix salicylic acid powder with alcohol until all crystals are dissolved and add Calendula Lotion (Tincture) and Camphor Spirits. Salicylic acid powder I recommend that you purchase from the website **www.drugsdepot.com**. The website offers several products of salicylic acid powder from different companies. The Camphor Spirits 2% widely sells in the pharmaceutical stores.*

Your investment to prepare microdermabrasion solution is going to cost somewhere around $20, but the solution will last you for quite a long time. You need to use it for any microdermabrasion treatments: anti-aging, acne, and hyperpigmentation or scar treatments.

➤ Step #5: Perform microdermabrasion.

Perform microdermabrasion according skin lines starting with forehead and moving down to the neck area.

Neck and eyes are first that starting to show sign of aging. If you perform microdermabrasion on mature skin, you have to treat these areas as well. For teenage acne facial, it is not necessary to work on the neck and eyes area.

➤ Step #6: Apply post-microdermabrasion mask.

The application of the post microdermabrasion treatment is very important step. Wipe the whole face with calendula tincture to clean and disinfect the skin. You can also add a high frequency massage on acne-affected areas. Follow with anti-bacterial mask. Review previous protocol for formulas and mask products recommendations.

➤ Step#7: Antibacterial moisturizer application.

Finish with an anti-bacterial moisturizer.

Everyone skin is a little different and sometimes it takes more than one type of treatment to get a good result. However, there is absolutely a solution for every acne patient. Persistence and dedication is the key. No one can fix the problem with one miracle product or one treatment. Properly done, anti-acne facials and the right skin care products have to work in synergy to provide relief for acne sufferers. And our goal as a skin care professionals is to give our clients the best knowledge and services that we can provide. We have the amazing ability to change the way they look and feel about themselves.

Chapter 5: Rosacea

To achieve excellence as a skin care professional you have to be able recognize the most common skin disorders and take appropriate action, by either advising client to seek medical professional help or if it is belongs to esthetician scope to perform skin treatment procedures. In the previous chapter, I introduced to you several methods of treatment for acne. This chapter is dedicated to another skin disorder, called rosacea (roz-ay-sha) that estheticians may see on their clients.

Rosacea is a very common benign skin disorder that affects many people worldwide. As of 2008, it was estimated to affect at least 14 million people in the United States alone. Rosacea (acne rosacea) is a chronic skin condition that unfortunately can last throughout someone's life and requires a specific skin care routine and lifestyle habits to keep symptoms under control. The symptoms tend to come and go. The skin may be clear for weeks, months, or years and then erupt again. Triggers, such as sun exposure, heat, extreme cold or strong wind, sauna, steaming rooms, or consumption of alcohol or coffee can worsen the condition and bring symptoms back.

The main symptoms of rosacea include red or pink patches, visible blood capillaries, small red bumps, red cysts, enlarged pores, excessive oil production, and multiple "so-called" black and whiteheads. It characteristically involves the central region of the face, causing persistent redness or transient flushing over the areas of the face and nose that normally blush — mainly the forehead, the chin, and the lower half of the nose. In women, the redness usually appears on the cheeks, nose, chin, and forehead in a "butterfly" pattern. Facial redness in men typically appears on the nose, although symptoms can appear on other areas of the face. In some cases, redness may also occur on the neck and upper chest.

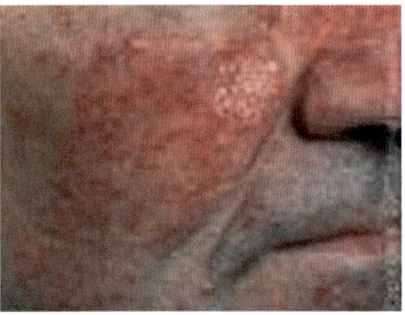

Typical Signs and Symptoms

The signs and symptoms of rosacea will vary, depending of the individual. However, most symptoms and signs include the following:

- Small pimples may occur on the red areas of skin or on the edges. The pimples are red and round bumps and they are different than acne pimples, which are blackheads or whiteheads.

- Broken or dilated capillaries on the face are called telangiectasia. These small, thin blood vessels look like a spider webs, and they usually appear on the cheeks.

- Swollen bumps on the nose in severe cases, mostly in men, called Rhinophyma. The nose is one of the first areas to be affected by Rosacea. It becomes red and bumpy and develops noticeable dilated small blood vessels. Left untreated, advanced stages of Rosacea can cause a growth of the nose, characterized by a bulbous, enlarged red nose and puffy cheeks. There may also be thick bumps on the lower half of the nose and the near cheek areas. Severe case of Rhinophyma can require surgical repair.

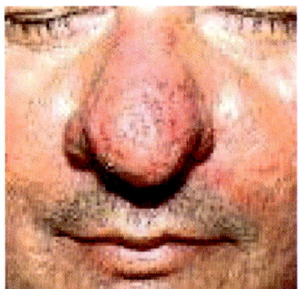

- Eye irritation with symptoms that include redness, dryness, burning, tearing, a gritty feeling, like that of sand in the eye, pinkeye (conjunctivitis), and swelling in the eyelid are also can be present. In some cases, vision may be blurry, but it is mostly in severe cases of this skin disorder. About half of the people with rosacea have some eye irritation.

Main roles in the development of rosacea play in the neurological disorder that creates the pathology of vascular system (excessive dilation of capillaries), inflammation of hair follicles (*Demodex*) and pathological changes in digestive tract and endocrine system. Inflammation of hair follicles, caused by microscopic skin mites, called Demodex, can contribute to this skin irritation. This is a mite that occurs naturally in the hair follicles of most adults, but in many people, these mites never cause a problem. But in certain health conditions, such as an impaired immune system, intense stress, and digestive tract problems, the mites can reproduce rapidly, causing hair follicles inflammation. The Demodex can mostly be found on oily skin that has abnormal sebum production that this small parasite "feeds" on.

Forms of Rosacea

There are several clinical forms of Rosacea. They include the following:

- *Erythematotelangiectatic Rosacea*
  Skin condition when skin has permanent redness (Erythema) and broken capillaries visible on surface of the skin

- *Papulopustular Rosacea*
  Skin condition with papullas (red bumps) and pussy pustules

- *Phynatous Rosacea*
  Skin condition with of Rhinophyma, an enlargement of nose

- *Ophthalmorosacea*
  Skin condition associated with red, dry and irritated eyes and eyelids

- *Steroid-induced Rosacea*
  Skin irritation caused by the use of topical or nasal steroids.

Most people with this skin disorder may not even know they have rosacea or that it is a diagnosable and treatable condition. When rosacea sufferers notice inflammatory papules on their faces, or lumpy-bumpy skin texture, they often treat these symptoms with harsh skin care products and topical medications that are supposed to help "smooth out" the skin. Certain treatments of bumps, uneven skin texture, and enlarged pores are often dangerous for rosacea clients and treatments like microdermabrasion, chemical peels have been reported to worsen the skin condition. Additionally, topical products like benzoyl peroxide, accutane, and retinoid can actually trigger Rosacea.

Procedures that are not recommended for people with Rosacea:

- Dermabrasion or microdermabrasion to treat enlarged pores, acne, wrinkles, or uneven skin texture
- Chemical peels of any kind
- Any form of UV light therapy
- Nose strips, mud masks, and buffer machines
- Skin suction or vacuum devices. These procedures are notorious for damaging micro vessels and may cause its breakage.
- Freezing of skin with liquid nitrogen (cryotherapy)
- Any scrubs or mechanical abrasion with harsh loofa
- Depilatories (chemicals that remove the hair)
- Electrolysis
- Waxing
- A facial performed by an esthetician that does not have experience working with clients who have rosacea

Treatment of Rosacea

Tips to Keeping Rosacea Under Control

By following the below tips, one can more easily keep their Rosacea symptoms under control.

- ➢ Avoid sun exposure by any means. Usage of sunblock or hat is essential.
- ➢ Avoid extreme hot like a sauna, steam room, or a hot bath. Avoid extreme cold and windy weather conditions as well.
- ➢ Stress reduction by controlling it with deep breathing, yoga, or other relaxation techniques.
- ➢ Limit spicy foods, alcohol, and hot coffee beverages.
- ➢ Avoiding any steroid drugs that can induce rosacea flair ups.
- ➢ Avoiding cosmetics and facial products that contain alcohol.
- ➢ Heavy exercise should be replaced with mild to moderate sport activities

Creams, lotions, foams, washes, gels and pads that contain various topical antibiotics, metronodazole, sulfacetamide, benzoyl peroxide, cortisone and retinoids are often prescribed by dermatologists to treat patients with rosacea. A slight improvement can be seen after few weeks of use, however, as I have mentioned above, these medicated products can cause of a thinning of the skin and flare-ups upon discontinuation.

Oral antibiotics have been a mainstay of rosacea treatment for years, and they tend to produce faster results than topical medication. But it can only work for up to several months before the bacteria become immune to the antibiotic, causing the antibiotic to lose its effectiveness. Besides, prolonged usage of oral antibiotics destroys intestinal healthy bacteria that can create serious health issues. There are many alternative treatments to help with rosacea skin problems, and with proper eating habits and proper skin care program the symptoms can be fairly well controlled.

To relieve the symptoms of Rosacea, one has a to start with an intestinal and liver cleansing program to detoxify the body. Healthy digestive track is the key to healthy skin. I believe that treating rosacea from the inside and from the outside can reduce it or even cure it. Many herbal-cleansing programs can help to get rid of toxins from the body and dietary changes may help to clear up the skin.

Skin care routine for people with rosacea has to include using mild cleanser specifically designed for sensitive skin and a soothing moisturizer with sun block of SPF30. Facial product should not burn, sting, irritate, or cause redness, in contrary it has to be very gentle and mild. One should wash their face with lukewarm water, avoiding harsh toners, astringents, scrubs, and facial loofas. Products that contain glycolic or lactic acid are also not recommended. My favorite choice for moisturizer is practically any moisturizer that is water-based with aloe vera gel. Greasy and heavy moisturizers can contain mineral oils that can aggravate rosacea symptoms.

Rosacea Treatment Protocol

For many years, I have been searching for a product that can safely and effectively relieve rosacea symptoms, and I have developed my own protocol for a facial designed for rosacea clients. It includes all basic steps of the facial but the products that have to be used are the key to a successful treatment. A facial can be a truly pampering experience for people who have rosacea; however the esthetician has to be aware that certain products can actually damage rosacea skin. If you feel confident to perform a facial for rosacea clients, make sure not to use any of these substances on their skin; alcohol, eucalyptus, fragrances, menthol, peppermint, or witch hazel. These ingredients are most likely to aggravate rosacea. It is also necessary to ask your client if she or he aware of any another ingredients or products that can aggravate the symptoms.

- Step #1: Cleanse.

    Cleansing with a mild cleanser for sensitive skin - I am suggesting Gentle Cleansing Gel from Raya Lab, Inc. It is specifically designed for dry and sensitive skin. The cleanser, based on aloe vera gel, is known for its healing and soothing properties. The aloe gel contains 96% water and 4% bio-stimulating agents that heal and regenerate skin.

- Step #2: Exfoliate.

    Remember, no exfoliation or steaming allowed while treating rosacea skin condition. So instead you can use soothing pre-extraction mask, which softens the comedones and diminishes erythema.

    Rosacea Exfoliating Mask Recipe

    To prepare the mask, you have to mix finely ground oatmeal (1 ounce) with Luke-warm distilled water. You can prepare ground oatmeal by grinding oatmeal flakes in a coffee grinder. Mix it all together to receive a "sour cream"-like consistency mask.

    Apply the mask on the face and neck with a spatula. Allow the mixture sit for 15 to 20 minutes, and then gently remove with damp washcloths. Wipe mask off with wet cellulose sponges.

- Step #3: Extract.

    If any pussy pustules or comedones need to be extracted (they are visible on the skin), remove it gently with soft tissue. Immediately after, saturate small cotton ball with Calendula Lotion and wipe the entire face. (Refer to the **Chapter 4: Acne vulgaris** for Calendula Lotion formula)

- Step #4: Apply a calming compress.
    Follow with calming compress. The compress can be prepared with boric acid powder or herbal infusion of sage, calendula, chamomile or valerian root.

    Boric Acid Calming Compress Recipe:

    Boric Acid power is available as an over- the-counter product at the drugstore.

Dissolve one teaspoon (5 g) of boric acid powder in 2 oz. of Luke-warm distilled water.
Saturate pre-cut gauze facial mask in prepared solution and apply it on whole face for 15-20 min.

Herbal Infusion Recipe:

A standard herbal infusion is prepared by adding 1 to 2 teaspoons of dried herb (or 2 to 4 teaspoons of fresh herb) to a cup of boiling water. Infuse for 10 minutes before straining. It's best to use a ceramic pot with a lid.

Or you can also use 1 to 2 teaspoons of herbs, adding a cup of cold water. Bring the mixture gently to a boil. Keeping it covered, simmer for about 10 minutes.

Decoction is the method of choice for bark and seeds. Valerian root should be boiled in the water for 10 min and steeped for 10 min. Cool off the infusion to room temperature and make compress with pre-cut gauze mask. Keep it for 15-20 min.

➢ Step #5: Follow with a non-contact high frequency treatment.

Follow with non-contact high frequency for 3-5 min. Put a small amount of medicated powder on the face and apply the glass tip, according to skin lines without touching the skin. Instead of medicated powder, you can use soothing formula from Raya Lab, Inc., called Aloe Vera Soothing Gel. It contains varieties of healing botanical extracts based on aloe vera gel. This product will comfort dry, chapped, and irritated skin.

➢ Step #6: Apply a soothing mask.

Apply Azulen Soothing Masque (Raya Lab, Inc.) for 15 min to constrict the pores and calm the skin. You can also prepare your own soothing mask, containing kaolin, zinc oxide, and aloe vera gel, mentioned above.

Mask with Aloe Vera and Kaolin Recipe

Mix equal part (one teaspoon) of kaolin clay and Aloe Vera gel. Add 1/4 teaspoon of zinc oxide powder.
Add a few drops of jojoba oil to provide a moisturizing effect to choppy, dry skin. Mix them all together to a creamy consistency.

The importance of jojoba oil in the treatment of Rosacea comes from its similarity to the natural restorative oil produced by the sebaceous glands in the dermal layer of skin. Jojoba oil is non-allergenic and will not clog the pores. Jojoba oil will help reverse damage to the epidermis caused by rosacea and also helps replace moisture lost, due to skin damage. It is beneficial for skin healing within the middle layer of the epidermis. Jojoba oil helps balance sebum excretion and helps normalize the moisture level in the dermal layer of skin.

➢ Step #7: Apply a protective moisturizer.

Lastly, remove mask with wet washcloth or cellulose sponges and apply protective moisturizer. Moisturizer should be light and non-oily to help retain hydration in the skin, but not at all greasy since grease can plaque the pores. It is also has to contain UVA and UVB sunscreen filters for enhanced skin protection. Moisturizer with sunscreen, based on aloe vera gel, is considered to be the best.

I prefer Azulen Day Cream from Raya Lab, Inc. It is formulated specifically for sensitive and irritated skin and provides instant moisture relief with long-lasting soothing effects. Another good moisturizer for oily, comedonic skin is Vitamin B Day Cream. This non-greasy, water-based, oil control formula can be used as a final step in oily or combination skin with rosacea. Vitamin B complex (Yeast Extract) helps to regulate oil gland secretion to reduce possibility of clogged pores, inflammations, and breakouts, associated with rosacea.

Telangiectasia

One of most common symptoms of rosacea is the dilated facial capillaries called *telangiectasia*. Leading skin care companies have been developing a product that may help to reduce this esthetically disturbing skin defect. One of the moisturizers contains Vitamin K, and it claims to provide relief from facial spider veins. However, studies show that the skin care product containing Vitamin K is not very effective.

I have discovered other ingredients that can really show great results for telangiectasia. It is rutin (Vitamin P) and natural silica. Rutin is a bioflavonoid and is found in many plants, fruits, and vegetables. The richest source is buckwheat and bee pollen, but it is also found in citrus fruits, black tea, and apples. Rutin has strong antioxidant properties and works as a blood capillaries strengthener.

Therefore, either taking as a supplement or added to the aloe vera based moisturizer, this bioflavonoid can significantly illuminate broken capillaries. The skin care company "Reviva" makes a cream containing rutin and other beneficial ingredients for varicose vein and spider veins. I also recommend to my clients with rosacea to take rutin as a supplement or bee pollen since it is also great source of rutin.

Silica is a mineral, or more properly silicon, is essential to keep bones, cartilage, tendons and artery walls healthy. It is present in onions, wheat, oats, millet, barley, alfalfa, and a variety of herbs like horsetail. Research shows that without sufficient amount of silica, the body cannot sustain optimum skin elasticity, strong hair, teeth, gums, bones, and walls of blood vessels. In addition, it is taking part in the synthesis of elastin and collagen, therefore, regenerating skin and the vascular walls. Taking Silica as a daily supplementation can help to reduce the appearance of spider veins and prevent capillaries from breakage. Many nutritional companies manufacture this supplement, and it can be found at any vitamin store.

Today, medical help is available that can control the signs and symptoms in severe rosacea cases. Some advanced skin care technology offers IPL (Intensive Pulse Light therapy) treatment for spider veins on the face. The IPL system was developed specifically for the treatment of vascular lesions, such as facial telangiectasia. The IPL therapy is centered on the removal of damaged and dysfunctional micro vessels and offers relief from the redness and flushing symptoms of Rosacea. The procedure has to be done by physician, dermatologist, or skin care professional under physician supervision. The IPL procedure corrects severe damages caused by rosacea when esthetic treatment does not provide the desirable effect.

Our goal as skin care professionals is to prevent it from happening. The earlier that a person is aware that she or he has rosacea, the greater the chances to have healthy looking skin by doing esthetic therapy, nutritional supplementation, and maintaining proper life style.

Chapter 6: Skin Aging

Aging is a complicated biological process that involves major changes of structure and function of human body. It affects all internal and the external organs, like our skin. Aging neck and face skin starts approximately at the age of 30 to 35 or even earlier for some individuals. With age, the body's metabolism and rejuvenating processes are slowing down and result major changes in the skin appearance. Our skin starts gradually losing its pink, healthy tone and its elasticity. The skin becomes dry, pale, and saggy. Numerous wrinkles start developing around the eyes ("crow's feet") then around the mouth, between eyebrows, and forehead.

Signs of Aging

Aging skin has many signs. Some of them are the following:

1. When we are young, the epidermal cells of our skin turn over about every 30 days. As we get older, the activity in the basal layer slows and cells start dividing much slower. By the age of 80, cells turnover takes twice as long as we were 30. As a result, the epidermal layers become thinner and more fragile.

2. The dryness of the skin appears, due to diminishing oil production by sebaceous glands. In men's skin, this process usually begins after the age of 80. However, women gradually produce less oil right after menopause. When hormonal changes occur, skin aging is an inevitable process, characterized by skin dryness, appearance of age spots, and wrinkles.

3. Changes in the connective tissue reduce the skin's strength and elasticity since collagen and elastin productions are significantly dropping. Collagen and elastin are the skin proteins responsible for elasticity, tone and texture. In youthful skin, collagen is firm, taut, and abundant, like a new mattress. As skin ages, collagen breakdown takes place, resulting in the appearance of fine lines and wrinkles.

4. With age, the number of pigment-containing cells (melanocytes) decreases and the remaining melanocytes tends to increase in size. Large pigmented

spots are known as age spots, liver spots, or lentigo may appear in sun-exposed areas. This process is called photo aging.

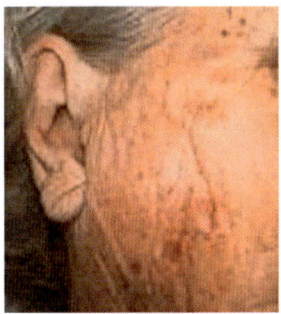

5. As skin ages, it loses it subcutaneous (fat) layer. In older skin, facial fat moves and resettles, changing the facial structure. The plumped up places on the face are losing its volume. Gravity pulls on both skin and the underlying fat, causing bags under eyes and sagging skin around the mouth and jaw line

6. The blood vessels become more fragile, so they are more likely to rupture and leak into the skin. This can lead to easy bruising, bleeding under the skin, cherry angioma (broken capillaries), "spider veins", and similar conditions.

7. The aging process involves not only skin itself, but beneath laying muscles and bones. In other words, as we get older, facial muscles are losing its firmness, becoming saggy, and losing its mass. The bone loss that gradually takes place and also contributes to an older looking skin.

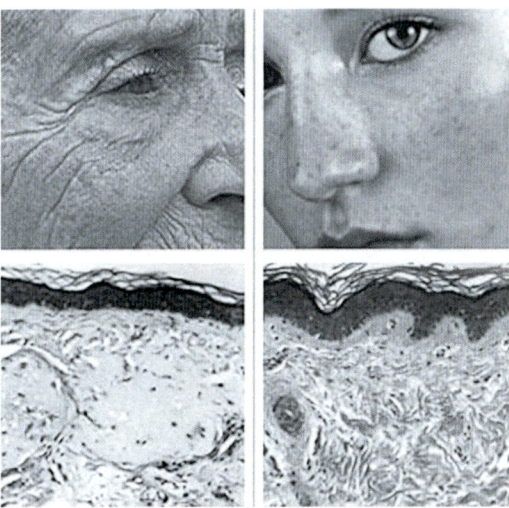

Effects of skin's aging mostly attribute to damage, caused by oxygen-free radicals, which affect every cell in our body, simply by virtue of the fact that oxygen is our principal metabolic fuel. Sun exposure can create an abundance of harmful free radicals that cause cell damage. Our hands, face, neck, and arms are the areas usually chronically exposed to the sunlight. As a result, these parts of the body, particularly face, are where aging of the skin shows up the most.

Skin protein, collagen, is particularly susceptible to free radical damage. And when this damage occurs, it causes collagen molecules to break down and then link back up again in wrong way. This process is known as cross-linking. Cross-linking collagen molecules are stiff and less mobile, which we recognize as sagging and wrinkled skin.

Skin for menopausal women often shows rapid aging due to drop in estrogen level. The estrogen is a female hormone that plays great part in the collagen metabolism. In the first years of menopause, estrogen level declines quickly and the amount of collagen decreases by as much as 2% per year.

Important factors that contribute to aging process are:

- Sun exposure -Sunlight is a major cause of the skin changes we think of as aging — changes, such as wrinkles, dryness, and age spots.
- First- or secondhand cigarette smoke
- Environmental toxins
- Poor diet
- Excessive alcohol consumption
- Stress
- Sleep deprivation
- Harsh soaps or mineral oil -based moisturizers

Today's cosmetic industry provides many effective methods to fight skin-aging processes that include antioxidant therapy, effective protection from UV exposure, hormone replacement therapy, varieties of esthetic skin care procedures, and advanced skin care products.

Most women by the age of 35 already start looking for professional skin care help to improve their skin complexion and to prevent future damage. No one wants to look old or prematurely aged. According my own statistics, 75% of my clients are seeking help with age related skin problems. No wonder, that the most common facial treatment is an anti- aging treatment. Among the most popular facial procedures are European anti-aging treatments with lymph-drainage massage, microdermabrasion, skin peels, ultrasound massage, micro-current facial lift, and LED (light emitting diode) therapy.

I customize my treatments according to skin needs and severity of skin damage. The benefits of professional skin treatments are tremendous, and I encourage my clients to do them on regular basis. For example, In France, Russia, and other European countries, facials are "must do" thing for most women. Historically, women from these cultures have been taking care of their skin, passing this good habit from mother to daughter.

The professional facial treatment provides an intensive skin cleansing by means of exfoliation and extraction. Facial massage helps to eliminate toxins from the head area and increase blood flow. The advanced facial techniques are offering superior treatment to eliminate free radicals, repairing sun damage, and encourage collagen production.

In this chapter, I want to share all of my most popular anti-aging techniques. I am including treatment protocols for you to review and use for your skin care services. I am also offering the most beneficial skin care formulations of creams and lotions that can be prepared by you to enhance the results of the treatments.

Generally speaking, I want to introduce you to my signature facials that I have developed during all the years that I have been practicing esthetics in the Ukraine and USA.

All anti- aging Facials include cleansing, exfoliation, extraction, massage, and application of the nourishing mask. Advanced anti-aging treatment, like microdermabrasion and peels, I will describe in separate chapters.

Let's begin with the most popular treatment: European Facial. This facial is the basic treatments that can be performed on all skin types. The procedure improves skin tone, restores skin balance, and provides deep moisturizing and nourishing effect. It includes exfoliation, extraction, lymph drainage massage, and facial mask application.

European Facial

> Step #1: Cleanse.

If you like using hot towels for your facials, you can start with hot towel application. This will softens the skin and opens the pores to facilitate skin cleansing. Proceed with the cleansing step, using appropriate cleanser. Usually the aging skin is dry, sensitive, or combination. In this case, you have to use cleanser for dry, normal, or sensitive skin.

If you are still looking for good professional line to enhance your performance, I can recommend you my favorite cleanser, manufactured by Raya Lab, Inc., Gentle Cleansing Gel. It is specially designed for normal, dry, and sensitive skin, and it cleans thoroughly, while moisturizing with natural botanical extracts. Based on aloe vera, it gently removes make-up and all other impurities. Perform light effleurage motion while spreading cleanser over the face and neck area. Remove the cleanser with damp cellulose sponges and follow with hot towel application.

The main purpose of cleansing is to remove make up, oil, and sweat impurities to provide initial skin stimulation by increasing blood and lymph circulation while exfoliating and preparing skin for further steps. It is important to follow proper cleansing techniques for best treatment performance. Once you learn this technique, it will stay in your memory and will take you no more than 3 min to go over whole face and décolleté.

For your knowledge, proper European Facial technique includes neck and the décolleté treatment. The neckline that exposes cleavage is called "décolleté" in current French language. This term has been known in worldwide professional esthetic terminology for several decades. Further in my book, I will use this term referring to the upper chest area.

In North America's esthetic procedures the décolleté area seems to be ignored by skin care professionals. The décolleté is exposed to the sun as much as face and starts showing sign of aging sometimes faster than face skin. It is essential to start caring for that area as much as we do face and neck.

How to Apply Cleanser

1. Warm up cleanser between moistened hands.

2. Approach face with both hands placing them on the temples.

3. Glide your hands down the sides of the face, then along the jaw line with fingers meeting at the chin. Place middle fingers over the upper lip keeping the remaining fingers under the chin. Glide back up to the temples.

4. Circle the eyes clockwise and glide down along the sides of the face. Then move your hand down to over neck and décolleté (upper chest),

around the shoulders and back up along the sides of the neck, stopping behind the ears.

6. With four fingers holding together, make circles down the neck, over décolleté toward shoulders, around shoulders, and back up the sides of the neck, stopping behind the ears.

7. Making the same circular motions, move along the jaw line toward the chin, back along the cheeks to upper lip and back toward ears.

8. Make small circles along nasal labial fold, gliding gently up the sides of the nose to the center of the forehead.

9. Glide back down over the bridge of nose making small circles down each side with the fingers of both hands, Glide back up to the center of the forehead.

10. Make circle motions along the forehead to the temples and back couple of times.

11. Circle the eyes three times, starting in between the eyebrows.

12. Effleurage forehead once with each hand.

13. With both hands glide down sides of the face stimulating cheeks with the fingers.

14. Glide down over the neck and décolleté, around the shoulder and back up to the temples.

15. Make circles on the temples with fingers.

You may also use this technique for the application of massage oils lotions. The method of application provides benefits for skin by increasing blood circulation, removing impurities, stimulating lymph system.

How to Remove Cleanser

1. Approach face at the temples with sponges in both hands.

2. With sponges, glide down the sides of the face, along jaw line to chin, down the front of the neck and over décolleté toward the shoulders, around the shoulders and back up the sides of the neck to the ears.

3. Effleurage décolleté and neck with sponges.

4. Flip over the sponges to clean sides of the face. Perform effleurage with alternating hands starting at the chin, working towards the side of the face. Repeat motion starting with upper lip.

5. Glide up the nasal labial fold and sides of the nose to the center of the forehead.

6. Clean nose area.

7. Circle eyes with sponger three times to remove residue of the cleanser.

8. Effleurage forehead once with each hand using sponges.

9. Glide down the sided of the face performing stimulating motion with sponges.

10. Glide down over the neck and décolleté, around the shoulders and back up to the temples.

> Step #2: Apply a toner.

Apply an appropriate toner or astringent to restore skin pH balance. The toner or astringent helps to remove the remaining traces of cleanser and make over. It restores pH balance and disinfects skin's surface.

> Step #3: Exfoliate.

I am sure that your professional skin care line has exfoliating product that you like to use. I personally like to use Bamboo Scrub manufactured by Raya Lab, Inc. This herbal exfoliating cream combines finely ground bamboo with jojoba beads and micro-fine French talc. It effectively removes dead cells of epidermis, lifts away dull, dry skin to improve texture of the skin.

After massaging skin with the scrub, remove it with damp washcloth or sponges. Follow with hot towel application to help open skin's pores before the extraction.

> Step #4: Extract.

Turn on steamer and steam face for 10 min and then perform an extraction. Use 3% hydrogen peroxide before the extraction and after to disinfect the skin surface (refer to the Chapter 4 for detailed extraction technique).

> Step #5: Apply an astringent.

After extraction apply astringent to disinfect the skin surface and close skin's pores. The astringent or toner can be diluted with distilled water and used as a facial spray. Spay the mixture over the face and let it to absorb.

Remove residue of moisture from the face with a clean tissue.

> Step #6: Perform an anti-aging massage.

Facial massage is the most important part of anti-aging treatment.

There are two types of anti-aging massages commonly used in European Facial technique: lymph-drainage and plastic massage. Duration of the massages should not last more than 15 min. (Refer to detailed description below.)

> Step #7: Apply a nourishing mask.

After massage, follow with nourishing mask application for 15-20 min. Remove mask with the water or damp washcloth. Apply appropriate moisturizer or sunblock if needed. (Refer to all formulas of anti- aging and nourishing masks further below in this chapter)

Lymph-Drainage Massage

To perform any cosmetic procedure and facial massage, an esthetician can greatly benefit from knowing detail facial anatomy and topography of the human head; otherwise, incorrect motion can harm the client and cause unpleasant sensations. Knowing of location of facial group of muscles and bones help accurately perform massage motion in accordance with important anatomical landmarks. It gives skin care specialists more confidence during the facial treatment and can even increase the effectiveness of their work.

Facial massage has incredible benefits for human skin and facial muscles since it has positive influence on the whole human organism. In the process of massage, there are involved the numerous nerve endings that provide stimulating or calming effect. For example, a gliding motion calms down the nerves and muscles, while a kneading motion stimulates it.

The anti-aging facial massage helps to rejuvenate, tone, and firm the skin and facial muscles. It improves color of the facial complexion and normalizes sebum production by oil glands. The duration of the facial massage depends on the skin condition, client age, and physical shape. Usually the lymph-drainage facial massage lasts around 15- 20 minutes, too long of a massage may cause feeling of fatigue and irritation.

The most popular facial massage for European Facial is the lymph-drainage anti-aging massage. Indications for this type of massage are dull, lack of tone, and elasticity skin. The massage facilitates skin rejuvenation processes and toxins removal from head area. This is of one of my favorite types of massages that I use for almost all age related skin problems.

There are some contra-indications for lymph-drainage massage as well as inflammatory or cystic acne, oily comedonic skin, seborrhea dermatitis, psoriasis, rosacea, atopic dermatitis, facial nerve damage, head traumas, or abundant facial hair.

The benefits of the lymph-drainage massage are superior compared to other anti-aging techniques, and it is one of the main parts of the European Facial.

It helps to:

* Minimize skin sagging and fine lines
* Release toxins and impurities
* Increase skin cells nourishment
* Normalize skin's moisture balance
* Release tension
* Balance oil production by sebaceous glands
* Increase nutrients absorption

Techniques of the massage are based on the theory of lymph-drainage that defines principals of all massages. The procedure includes superficial massage, facial muscles massage, and massage of facial nerves. All motions have to be performed in sequence, smoothly moving from one step to another and in accordance with skin lines.

There are five common massage motions involved in it; effleurage, friction, kneading, percussion, and vibration. The main purpose of effleurage and frictions is to increase blood and lymph circulation. Kneading is the main method to stimulate facial muscles and facilitate muscle toning. Vibration motion helps to stimulate facial muscular-nervous system to increase metabolic and regenerative processes.

For better performance, it is necessarily to use massage oil or massage cream.

Lymph-Drainage Massage Protocol

> Step 1: Apply lotion.

Apply massage cream or massage oil, according facial skin lines. Refer to the cleanser application technique to spread lotion on client's face.

If you prefer to use massage oils, here is fabulous formula that you can prepare mixing several oils together.

Massage Oil Recipe

Almond oil	2.5 oz
Jojoba oil	0.5 oz
Wheat germ oil	0.5 oz
Avocado oil	0.5 oz
Sunflower oil	0.5 oz
Olive oil	0.5 oz
Vitamin E oil	0.5 oz
Aloe Vera gel	2 oz
Glycerin	1 oz

Above-mentioned ingredients can be found at your local health food store or pharmacy store.

> Step 2: Effleurage.

Effleurage is the gliding stoke that performs according facial massage lines.

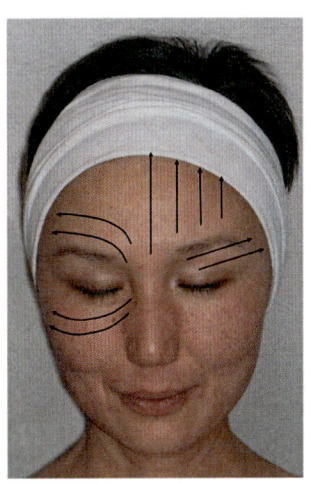
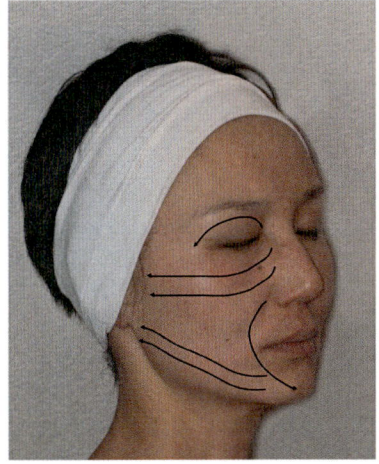

It has to be done with four fingers holding together. Repeat each round 3 times. With the back of the hands gently glide across the forehead.

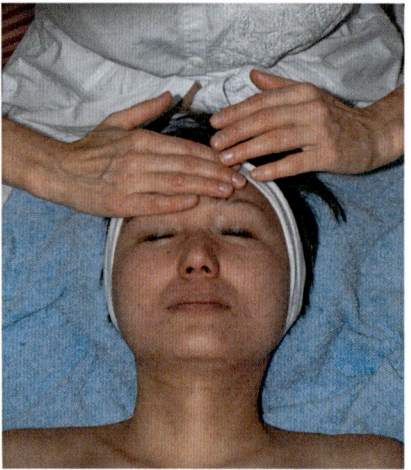

The gliding stroke around the eyes has to start counter clock wise from beginning of eyebrow to the inner hollow of the eye. Use index and middle finger only to perform orbital effleurage. Use entire palm of both hands to effleurage cheeks, jaw-line, and chin.

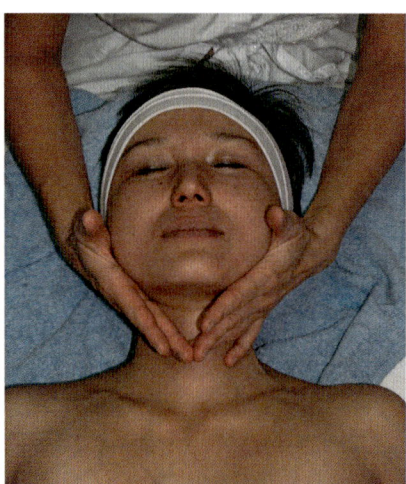

Use fingers tips of both hands to glide around mouth.

Then follow with the lymph-drainage stroke. The lymph-drainage is the gliding motion that performs in the beginning of massage and between each steps of it. Please, refer to the picture for proper hand position of lymph-drainage effleurage.

Fix the thumbs of both of your hands on the nose bridge, while holding your palms under the chin. Glide four fingers of both hands, holding tight towards the ears area. Then glide along the sides of the neck down to clavicle bone. Perform this motion 3-4 times to stimulate lymph-drainage.

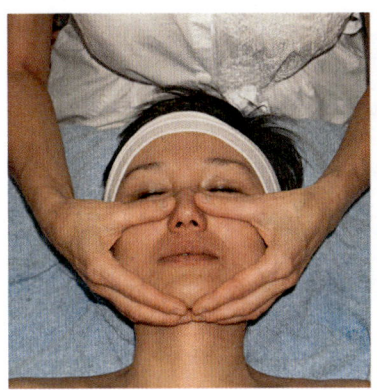 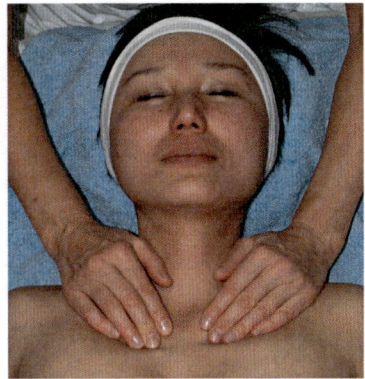

Perform effleurage one more time of entire face as described above. Finish this step with lymph-drainage gliding stroke again. Repeat 3 times.

- Step #3: Perform friction strokes.

Friction motions begin with the circular friction strokes of the décolleté area slowly heading up to the chin area. Make sure your fingers are moving gently without pulling the skin.

Perform spiral friction strokes using fingers tips, massaging entire face according skin lines. Repeat each area 3 times.

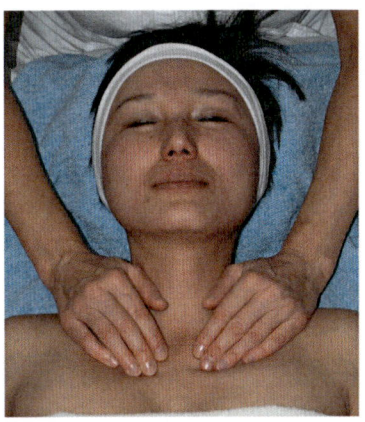 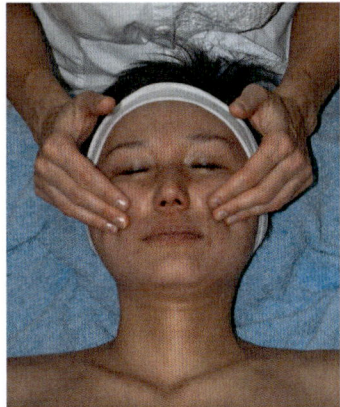

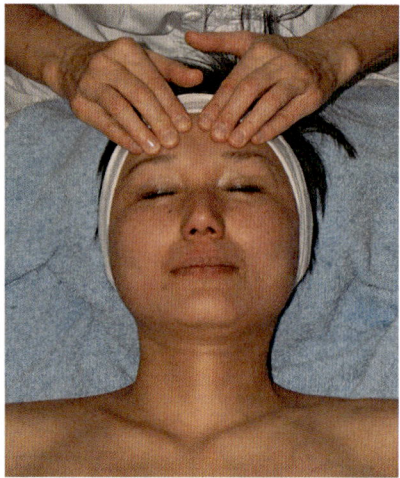

Then move again to the base of the neck and do spiral friction strokes heading up to the jaw line. Slight pressure should be applied while massaging the jaw muscles. Repeat 3 times.

To massage nose muscles use thumbs of both hands keeping palms under the chin and gently massage nose muscles in circular motions.

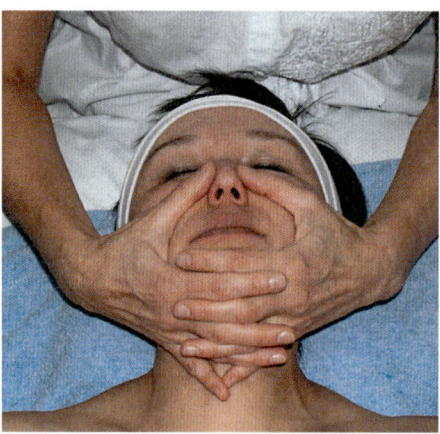

Then move to the eye area to perform small circular friction strokes, starting from the top of eyebrows, moving counterclockwise wise to the inner corners of the eyes. (Repeat 3 times.)

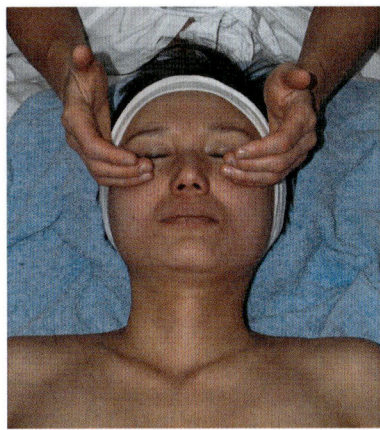

On the forehead, friction stroke starts from top of eyebrows moving to hairline. Slight pressure may apply to feel forehead muscles. (Repeat 3 times.)

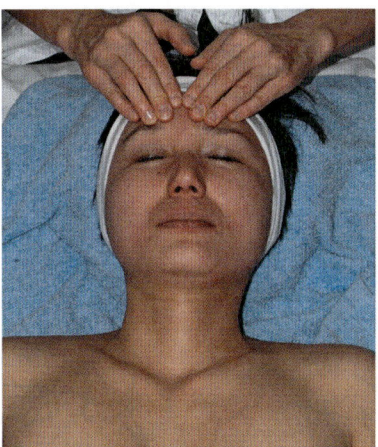

Finish this step with lymph-drainage stroke. Repeat 3 times.

➢ Step #4: Perform kneading.

With knuckles of both hands, perform kneading strokes. Begin circular kneading motions from the décolleté area to the base of the neck and jaw line.

Follow each step with kneading all facial muscles group: jaw, cheeks, orbital, forehead, and temples. Repeat each motion 3 times.

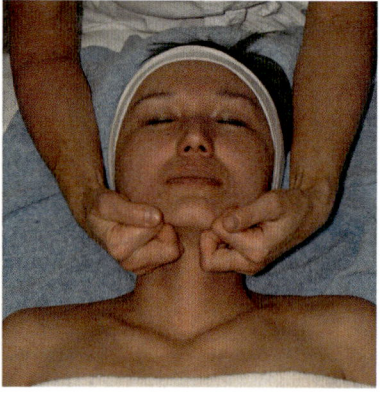

Finish the step with lymph-drainage stroke, repeating 3 times.

- Step #5: Use a percussion motion.

Using the tips of the fingers conduct spiral "staccato" motion, according skin lines, moving up the base of the neck to the jaw lines and from cheeks toward forehead. Repeat twice for the whole face.

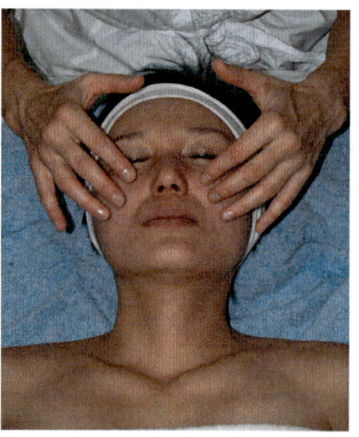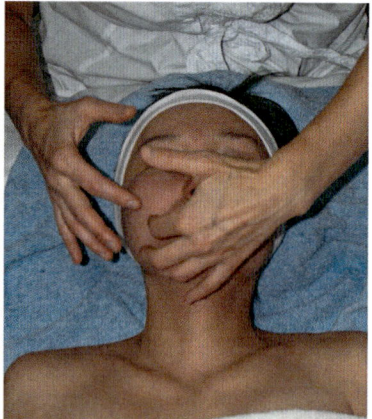

Finish this step with lymph-drainage stroke, repeating it 3 times.

- Step #6: Vibrate.

Vibration step has two parts. Gently pinch each piece of skin between index and thumb, starting from the base of the neck moving toward jaw line. Move along the skin lines to perform massage on jaw line, cheeks, around the mouth, orbital (eye) area, and forehead.

On the forehead, strokes should start between the eyebrows, moving toward hairline.

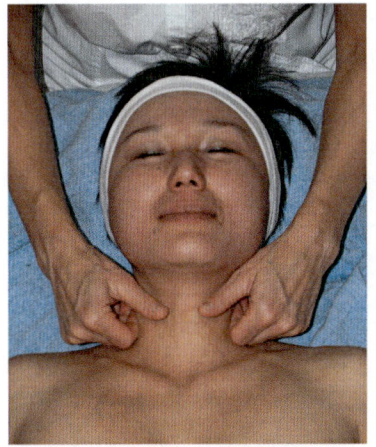
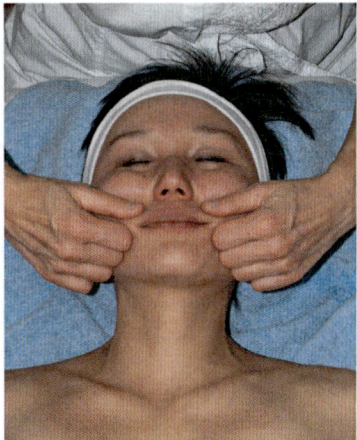
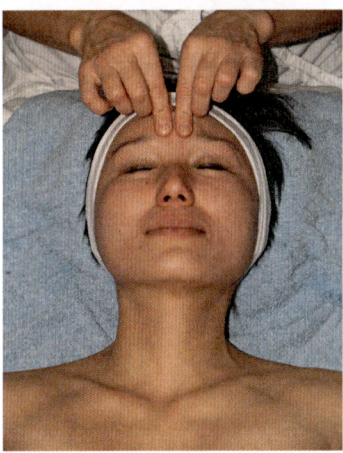

Perform second step of the vibration by pinching skin between index fingers and thumbs and add slight vibration to each pinch. Start with the base of the neck moving toward to jaw line. Follow with entire face, according to skin lines. Repeat vibration stroke three times to each facial muscles group.

Finish this step with the lymph-drainage stroke (3 times).

➢ Step #7: Perform chin kneading.

People with a double chin need extra work around chin area. With knuckles of both hands perform kneading the tissue under the chin for 2-3 min finishing with gliding stroke.

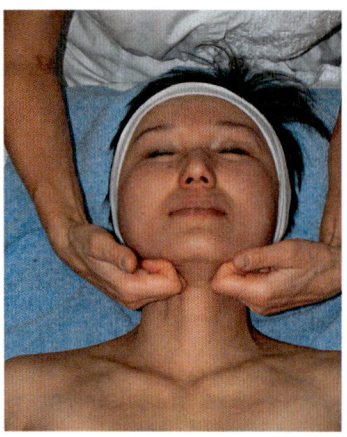 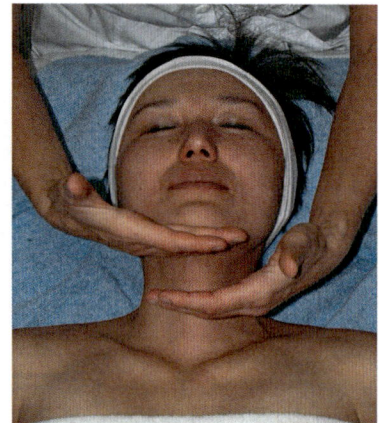

➢ Step 8: Repeat effleurage.

At the end of massage, perform gliding stroke (refer to the first step) starting from décolleté and up.

Plastic Facial Massage

There is another type of anti-aging massage that I want you to be familiar with. It is very effective facial massage technique that stimulates facial muscles and provides mini face-lift effect. It is superior facial massage that has strong benefits for flabby and lack of tone aging skin.

This type of massage has the same indications and contra-indications as lymph-drainage massage. But, in contrary with lymph-drainage massage, you do not need use massage cream or oil. It performs over medicated powder or Aloe vera gel.

The technique involves 4 different strokes: effleurage, kneading, percussion, and vibration. All strokes should be performed with the back of the hands by applying different pressure to the different groups of facial muscles.

➢ Step #1: Effleurage.

Begin with gliding stroke (effleurage) using back of your palms gently follow along the facial skin lines. Every facial line has to be effleurage three times, finishing with the slight fixation.

Start from the middle of forehead, moving toward the temples. Then glide from the middle of the nose toward the cheekbones. Lastly, glide from the middle of the chin along the jaw-line toward the ears.

Do not forget the neck and décolleté. Perform effleurage, starting from the clavicle bone toward jaw and chin.

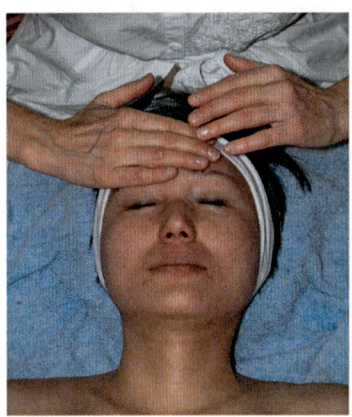 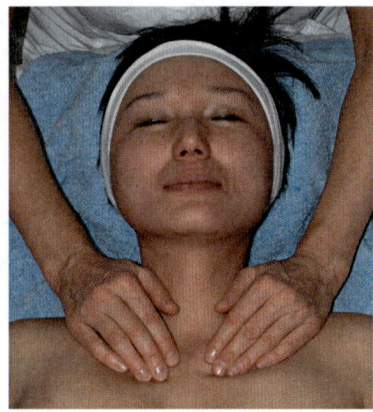

> Step #2: Perform kneading strokes.

Perform circular kneading strokes, according to facial lines. The motion has to be strong and rhythmic, gently pressing skin to the bone. Feel every muscle group that your fingers touch, while performing a circular kneading motion.

The kneading step has two rounds. First round is a circular kneading motion with the tips of four fingers of both hands, while slightly pressing skin to the bone. Second round is also circular kneading motion but with the knuckles of the fingers.

Start this step from the forehead moving toward the temples. Then proceed from the inner corner of the eyes toward the top of the ears. Next line begins from the nostrils and goes to the middle part of the ears. Then move your hands from the middle of the chin along the jaw-line toward the earlobe. Each facial line repeats 3 times, finishing each facial line with slight fixation. Lastly, massage neck muscles, starting from clavicle bone, moving upward towards the jaw-line.

The kneading step is the most important step of this type of facial massage. It brings blood flow to the muscles and improves its tone and firmness, while increasing its volume.

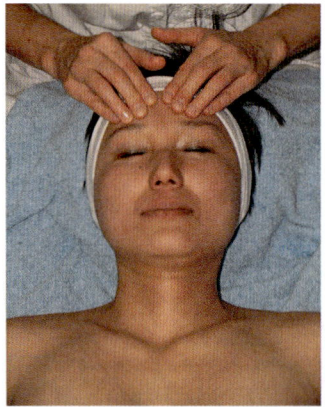
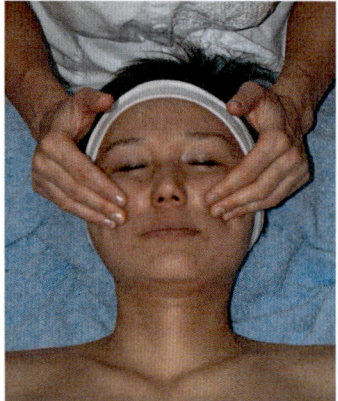

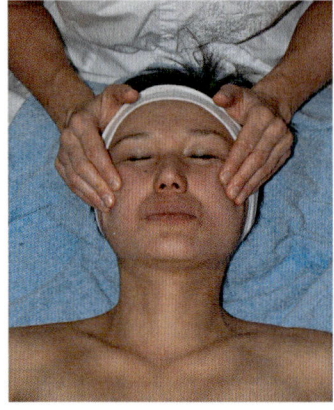

Please, refer to the pictures below for positioning your hands, while performing circular kneading with knuckles.

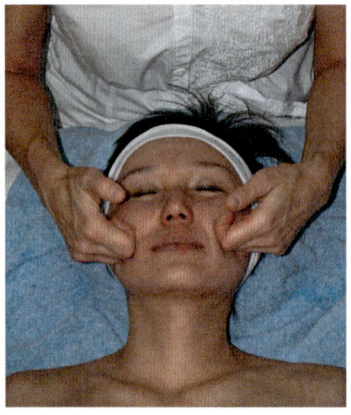
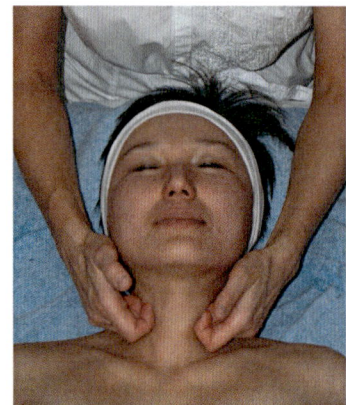

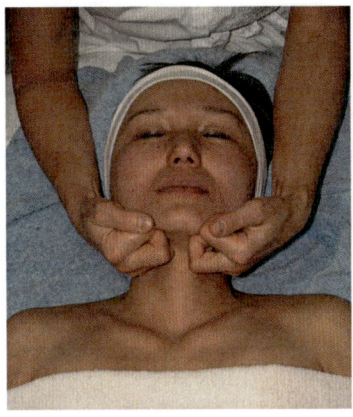

The kneading with the knuckles is an effective way to stimulate acupressure points of the face. Stimulation of these points gives additional benefits to the plastic massage in order to provide face-lift effect.

Press skin to the bone with the knuckle of index finger and gently stimulate the point in circular clockwise motion. Duration for each point is 10 -15 seconds. Refer to the diagram below to locate facial acupressure points.

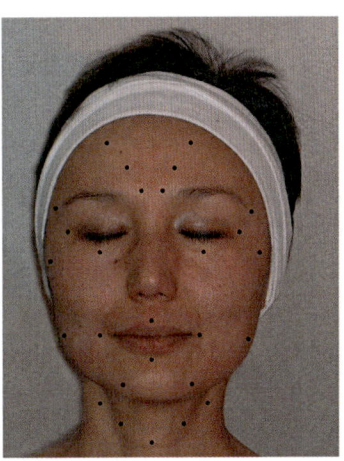 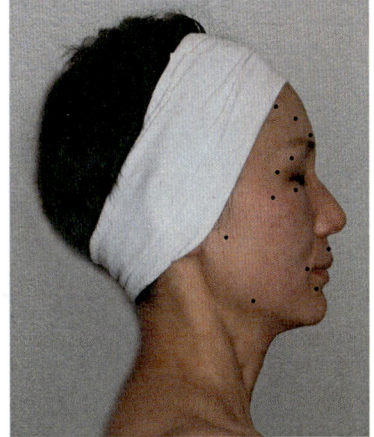

➢ Step #3: Perform a percussion motion.

Using only tips of the four fingers conduct spiral "staccato" motion (percussion) according to the skin lines, starting from forehead and heading towards the base of the neck. Repeat twice on the entire face.

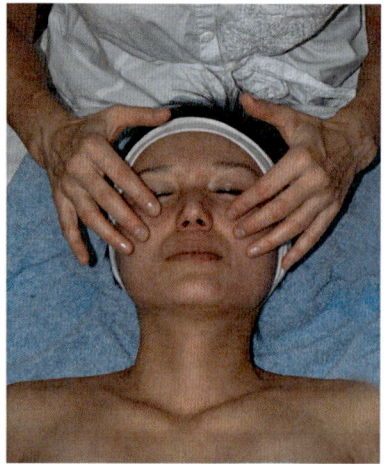

➤ Step #4: Vibrate.

Lastly, perform vibration movements by pressing and vibrating facial muscles with all fingers of both hands. Repeat this motion twice for the entire face and neck area.

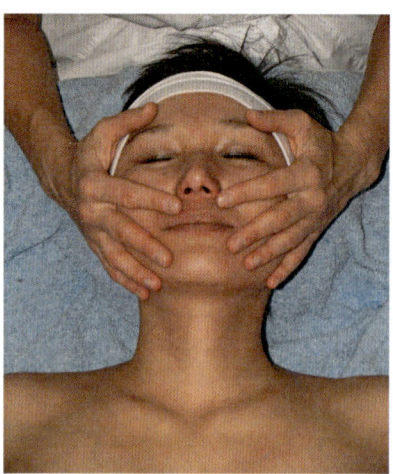

➤ Step #5: Effleurage.

Light effleurage is the final stage of the plastic massage. Perform it in the same manner like in step one.

Cosmetic Masks and Lotions

Facial mask application is an important step of all esthetic treatments, including acne, anti-aging, microdermabrasion, etc. The range of masks varies from anti-inflammatory and disinfecting to tightening, calming, and nourishing.

Classification of Masks

There are many different types of facial masks. And they can be classified in the following ways:

- Based on the level of action, they can be epidermal and trans-epidermal.

- Based on type of skin, they can be for oily, dry, and normal skin.

- Based on action, they can be cleansing, exfoliating, anti-bacterial, moisturizing, nourishing, regenerative, firming, and tightening.

- Based on the shape, they can differentiate on creamy masks, gel–masks, paste masks, and powder masks.

Anti aging cosmetic masks should provide deep nourishment, regenerative and moisturizing effect. For their preparation, you can use different cosmetic ingredients, including natural and synthetic source. As a base for masks, you can use vegetable oils, bee wax, cacao butter, lanolin, paraffin, glycerin, lecithin, gelatin, clay, oatmeal, talk, zinc oxide, etc.

Active substances masks may include complex of bioactive ingredients like vitamins, herbal extracts, hormones, lipids, essential oils, aloe vera, and more.

The information in this chapter reveals numerous formulas of treatment masks and lotions that are proven to give desirable results. All preparations are based on either fresh ingredients from your kitchen or pharmaceutical over-the-counter ingredients.

Masks (homemade or otherwise) should stay on the skin for 15-20 minutes. It is the optimum time frame that skins needs to absorb all "good stuff" from the facial masque.

Meal masks should be prepared right before the treatment, and they can be stored in the refrigerator for day or two.

Nourishing Masks from Fresh Ingredients

One of the most highly effective masks can be prepared from fresh fruits and vegetables since they are the best source of vitamins, fats, and antioxidants.

For example, egg yolk has sufficient amount of Vitamin A and other vitamins and can be used as a source for other nourishing agent like lecithin. If you choose any cosmetic product lecithin is one of the main ingredients listed on the label. Its popularity based on excellent emulsifying properties and ability to hold water. Besides, lecithin has sufficient amount of phospho-lipids that provide deep moisturizing effects for the skin.

Lecithin Mask

Natural Lecithin mask is a nourishing treatment for normal and dry skin. Made from egg yolk, it contains natural lecithin (the most effective natural lipid) and Biotin (vitamin B). Added to masks, it delivers deep nourishing properties to dry and sun damaged skin.

You can make the lecithin from egg yolk in few easy steps. Separate 4 egg yolks from egg whites. Beat egg yolks with the mixer for 15min. until they double in size. Add to mixture 1 oz of castor oil and one teaspoon of glycerin. Beat again for 15min. Store the ready-to-use lecithin in the refrigerator and use it for your treatment as a base for any nourishing meal masks.

> *Lecithin Mask #1 Recipe*
>
> *1 teaspoon of lecithin*
> *Few drops of extra virgin olive oil*
> *Few drops fresh squeezed lemon juice.*
> *Apply fresh prepared mixture on the skin for 15-20 min. Remove with warm water or damp washcloth.*
>
> *Lecithin Mask #2 Recipe*
>
> *Mix equal parts (one teaspoon) of honey, lecithin, lemon, and cucumber juice. Apply for 15-20 min on whole face and neck. Remove with water or damp washcloth.*

Egg Whites Mask

Egg whites are pure protein, and can be applied directly to the skin. It greatly tightens the skin pores while it dries.

Honey Mask

When added to any mixture, it provides excellent skin stimulation effect. It can be used for dull and dry skin to increase blood circulation and increase blood circulation to improve color of the complexion.

Nourishing Mask Recipe for Dry, Sun-Damaged Skin

Beat one egg yolk with mixer for 10 min and add 1 teaspoon of honey. Apply mixture on the whole face and neck for 30 min. Wash with water and damp washcloth

Oatmeal Mask

Oatmeal has great cleansing properties, and, in addition, its gives gentle bleaching effect.

Cleansing, Soothing, and Nourishing Mask

1 teaspoon of fine ground oatmeal (I recommend using coffee grinder to grind oatmeal or dry herbs.)
1/2 teaspoon of honey
1 teaspoon of Aloe Vera gel
1 egg yolk
1/2 teaspoon of lemon or orange juice
This mask has great benefits for dull congested and aging skin.

Herbal Mask with Oatmeal and Jojoba oil

Combine equal part (1 teaspoon) of fine ground oatmeal, jojoba oil, wheat germ oil and avocado oil. Add a few drops of Vitamin E oil and lemon essential oil. The mask has moisturizing and nourishing properties for dry skin.

Cucumber Mask

Cucumber is known for its soothing and toning properties. It can be mixed with another ingredient like alum to reach excellent tightening pores effect.

Avocado Mask

Avocado can be added to any nourishing mask for dry skin. It works well when mixed with a few drops of fresh lemon juice and one teaspoon of extra virgin olive oil.

Avocado and honey mixed together are a particularly great moisturizing combination.

Aloe Vera and Avocado Mask after microdermabrasion.

Mix half of avocado with fresh aloe vera gel (from plant) and add few drops of fresh squeezed lemon juice. Mix well and store it the refrigerator.
You can use this mask for three days each time adding few drops of fresh lemon juice. This mask is excellent calming treatment after microdermabrasion.

Other Excellent Ingredients

Bananas are great for any toning mask since they have some tightening properties as well.

Pineapples are abundant in natural enzymes and Vitamin C. Added to the masks or just itself provides exfoliating action and, therefore, protects the skin from aging.

Papaya also has natural enzymes and works as an aid to remove dead cell and softening the skin.

Lemon is one of the strongest natural bleaching substances, due to citric acid content. It is also provides sufficient amount of Vitamin C in ascorbic acid form.

Oranges are one the important source of Vitamin C in it natural and available form. It can be mixed to any anti-aging mask to stimulate collagen production.

Plain yogurt or sour cream is excellent source of lactic acid that works like an exfoliator and skin brightener. It also contains animal fat that helps for skin lubrication. I use it as a base for many nourishing masks. For example, you can mix it with banana, avocado, and add few drops of lemon or orange juice. This composition has anti-aging properties for dry and sun-damaged skin.

Nutritional yeast, not to be confused with brewer's yeast, is packed with the B-complex Vitamins and proteins. B Vitamins are very important to maintain healthy and acne-free skin. Nutritional yeast can be used for cosmetic purposes to treat acne and acne prone skin.

Mask with Nutritional Yeast for Oily Skin.

Mix one tablespoon of nutritional yeasts with 1 tablespoon of 3% hydrogen peroxide. Use for oily skin with numerous comedones.
For dry skin, mix one teaspoon of nutritional yeast with one teaspoon of olive oil.

Herbal Masks

It is not a secret that herbs are widely used in the skin care industry. A majority of high-end cosmetic companies have been including herbal extracts in their formulas, due to the unbeatable benefits for the skin. I use several herbs in my formulas, preparing them as herbal infusions, herbal tinctures, or herbal masks.

To prepare an herbal mask, take finely ground herbs and add boiling water. Let it steep for 5-10 minutes. Squeeze the water out of the herbal mixture and spread the remainder on the face. Cover with wet gauze or warm towel. Duration of the application is about 15-20 min. Remove the mask and follow with appropriate moisturizer.

Herbal Mask for Congested and Sensitive Skin

Mix equal parts (1 teaspoon) of dry herbs, like chamomile, sage, oak bark, nettle, horsetail and St. John's Wort. Grind them in coffee grinder, and steep it in boiling water for 10-15 min. Squeeze water out of the herbal mixture and apply it on the face. Cover with the pre-cut gauze mask or warm wet towel.

Chamomile: Added to the mask provides an excellent calming and soothing effect.

Peppermint: has a cooling, soothing, and antiseptic action. This plant is rich in Vitamins A and C.

Sage leaves: have anti microbial, antiseptic and slight astringent properties.

Calendula: these flowers are my favorite herb for acne treatment. This miracle herb has been praised by herbalists for decades for every imaginable injury and damage to skin tissue, including burns, sunburns, eczemas, cuts, abrasions, pustules, lesions, and chapped skin. In my book, I refer to the Calendula tincture that I used in almost all of my treatments. Review Chapter 4, where I give the details of Calendula tincture preparation.

Comfrey leaves: these have the ability to heal the wounds, due to natural allantoin, carotene, and mucco-polysaccharides.

Horsetail: this herb is very high in natural silica. As I mention in Chapter 3, silica is one of the bio elements that is involved in keratin and collagen production. It helps to fight wrinkles and strengthen weak capillaries of the cupreous skin.

Hyssop extract: is used to treat skin irritations, burns, bruises, and cold sores, due to its healing ability.

Ginseng root: is widely known as an excellent tonic and rejuvenator. It has been used in creams, gels, tonics, and masks as anti- wrinkle agent.

Lavender flower: Famous lavender essential oil can be added to any lotion as a fragrance. Besides, added to moisturizers, it enhances antiseptic and anti-inflammatory action for acne treatments.

Stinging nettle: contains proteins, amino acids, vitamins, and minerals and can be used as aid for anti aging treatments. I use nettle herbal infusion for nourishing masks as a collagen production accelerator.

Oak bark: is mostly used as herbal infusion for toners and astringents, due to very strong tightening properties.

St. John's Wort: this herb is very popular in Europe due to its soothing and healing properties. Can be used as an astringent for oily and acne prone skin. Oil or tincture can be added to any cream or lotion for additional healing benefits.

Nourishing Masks and Creams

Plastic Hot Mask (Paraffin Mask)

This is an effective treatment for extremely dry skin. The mask is designed to seal the moisture into the skin and enhance the benefits of moisturizing cosmetic substances applied under the mask. It helps to hydrate, nourish, and stimulate the skin. The Paraffin Facial is an instant "fix" for dehydrated and overly stressed dull complexions.

The hot mask is not recommended after extraction since pores will remain open and become more susceptible to bacteria. However, it should be used right along with anti-aging lymph-drainage massage, since the treatment enhances skin decongestion and toxins removal.

Paraffin Mask Recipe

Pure professional grade facial paraffin 2oz (60gr)
Bee wax 1oz (30gr)
Cacao butter 2oz (60gr)
Almond oil 2oz (60gr)

Place all ingredients in small melting pot or wax warmer. Heat until the mixture completely melts, while constantly stirring. Take it from melting pot and test the temperature on your wrist to make sure the mask is not very hot. Use facial brush for mask application and begin to apply starting with the forehead. Wait at least three seconds before applying another layer. For best results, apply at least three layers. Cover the whole face with a hot towel leaving nostrils uncovered. Duration of the application 15-20 min. Remove cooled off mask with wet cloth and follow with an appropriate moisturizer.

This mask can also be used as a post-acne treatment to diminish acne spots and scars. Never use this mask on inflamed and acute acne skin conditions! Others skin conditions to not use this type of treatment on are: nodulecystic acne, rosacea, couperose skin, and hypertrichosis, or those with high blood pressure, claustrophobia, and bronchial asthma.

Besides of my own formulas, I also recommend varieties of nourishing masks offered by Raya Lab, Inc. My favorites are Placental Skin Recovery Masque, Natural Lecithin Masque, Collagen Treatment, Azulen-Paraffin, and Seaweed Fortifying Masque. For your convenience, these masks come in the salon size containers and retail size jars, as well, to offer it to your customers.

Lanolin Cream

Lanolin cream *is an* excellent heavy moisturizer that can be used for extremely dry skin or as an "after-microdermabrasion" healing cream. It is a unique formula that cannot find an alternative in any skin care lines. This formula provides an instant fix for dry and sun-damaged skin.

Lanolin Cream

Bee wax 2 oz (60 g)
Liquid lanolin 2oz (60g)
Cacao butter 1oz (30 g)
Almond oil 2 oz. (60 g) / (substitute 2 ounce almond oil with 2 ounce of jojoba oil)
Distill water 1 cup (236 g) or more if needed

Combine bee wax, lanolin, and cacao butter in small metal pot and heat it on low heat (70-73 C) until it melts. Remove mixture from the stove and slowly start adding oil, while constantly stirring with the mixer. Then gradually begin adding water stirring well. Mixture is going to cool off, and it will tend to get harder. Add more oil to receive a creamy consistency. Let it cool off completely and check the texture. If it is too runny, you can add more water; if it too hard, you can add more oil. This is a basic lotion, and you can add bio-active ingredients to it. For example, a few drop of Vitamin E, A, and D will enhance moisturizing properties of the cream. Also you can add any essential oil to add pleasant scent to it and any of the plant oils for deeper nourishment (like carrot oil, rose hips oil, avocado oil, etc.). There is no end to your creativity.

Aloe Vera Gel and Jojoba Oil

Personally, I like to add jojoba oil or jojoba butter. They are excellent substances for dry and sensitive skin. You can also replace water with aloe vera gel or mix it with equal parts of distilled water. The formulation can be used as a massage cream for anti-aging lymph-drainage massage. For massage cream, you can make it a little more liquid, adding more oils like sunflower, olive, wheat germ, etc.

Aloe Vera Moisturizer for Oily Skin

This contains aloe vera and can be easy prepared at your studio or salon.

Cacao butter	2 oz (60 g)
Lanolin	2.5 oz (75 g)
Honey	2 oz (60g)
Glycerin	1 oz (30 g)
Almond oil	2.5 oz (75g)
Olive oil	2.5 oz (75g)
Aloe Vera gel (pure)	6 oz (180g)
Distilled water	6 oz (180 g)

To make this preparation, simply combine the first four ingredients in small pot and heat it on small flame until all ingredients are melted. Gradually, add oils, then add aloe gel, and finally add water, while stirring the mixture with the mixer. As soon as the right consistency is achieved, store it in cool and dry place. Do not keep it in the refrigerator to prevent separation. If separation occurs, stir the whole mixture again.

Jojoba and Aloe Day and Night Cream

This is an alternative formula for dry and sensitive skin, prone to redness and irritation.

Jojoba Butter	1 oz (30 mg)
Jojoba oil	2 oz (60 mg)
Bee wax	1 oz (30 mg)
Cacao butter	1 oz (30mg)
Vitamin E oil	1/2 oz (15 mg)

Aloe Vera Gel   2 oz (60mg)
Glycerin   1 oz (30mg)
Distill water   3 oz or more if needed (approx. 100- 150 ml)

The method of preparation is the same as formula above.

Custom Blending

Custom blending allows the esthetician to customize products to the client's individual needs.

There can be another choice to get your custom blend product. Raya Lab, Inc. offers a variety of botanical extracts, super nourishing oils, vitamins, minerals, and seaweed extracts that permit skin care professionals to choose the product that suits to the clients skin type. With the incorporation of this approach to skin care, the esthetician acquires new skills and develops a reputation of being an expert and a professional.

In today's esthetic market, many skin care companies are manufacturing varieties of anti-aging products for salon treatments. A vast amount of them claim to contain some type of "magical ingredient" that promises it will take away or prevent wrinkles. The cost of these magical creams is ridiculously high, but it's not because of the expansive ingredients. Believe me; the ingredients have absolutely nothing to do with the prices that those companies charge for the product. All professional products are overpriced, due to market demand, since skin care professionals are always looking for the greatest product to increase effectiveness of their services. An advantage of custom blending lies in the ability of keeping up-to-date with the newest trends in skin care without having to continuously invest in numerous, different lines of cosmetics. Seems like every year professional products become more and more expensive, due to the newest, highly effective ingredients, like ceramides, peptides, collagen, elastin, etc. When new ingredients appear on the market, magazines and television immediately educate and influence the retail customer of the benefits of using a product with such components. Custom blending allows you to simply add any of these new ingredients to the basic product that is appropriate to an individual's skin type.

In conclusion, creating your own product for you customers is less costly, gives you the opportunity to put yourself ahead of the competition, and demonstrates an exceptional quality of a professional approach the client's expectations and demands.

Chapter 7: Hyperpigmentation

Hyperpigmentation is a common, usually harmless, condition in which patches of skin become darker in color than normal surrounding skin. The mechanism of excessive pigment deposits involves overproduction of melanin by hyper functional melanocytes, which are located in the epidermal and dermal layers of skin. Age or "liver" spots or freckles are common forms of *hyperpigmentation,* and they tend to occur when melanin-producing cells, a melanocytes, are damaged by UV radiation. These small, darkened patches are usually found on the hands and face or other areas frequently exposed to the sun, and they are referred to by doctors as a *"solar lentigo"*. *Solar lentigo* is the medical term for a freckle. Freckles are particularly common in people of fair complexion on upper-body skin areas, like cheeks, arms, and upper shoulders.

Melasma or chloasma spots are similar in appearance to age spots, but they are larger areas of darkened skin that appear most often as a result of hormonal changes. Pregnancy, for example, can trigger overproduction of melanin that causes the "mask of pregnancy" on the face and on the abdomen, or less commonly on other areas. Women who take birth control pills may also develop hyperpigmentation because their bodies undergo similar kinds of hormonal changes that occur during pregnancy. Melasma consists of dark brown, sharply emarginated symmetric patches of hyperpigmentation on the face (usually on the forehead, temples, and cheeks). Melasma is more prevalent and lasts longer in people with dark skin.

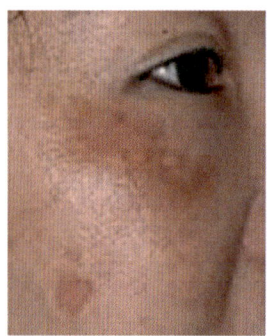
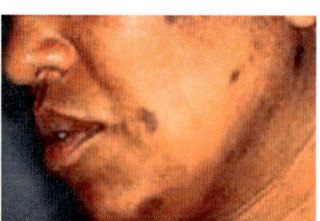
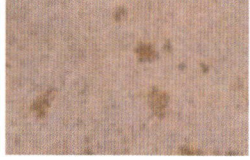

Other than sun exposure and hormonal changes, other factors that cause hyperpigmentation can be certain prescription drugs, liver damage, thyroid problems, acne vulgaris, atopic dermatitis, insect bites, psoriasis, mechanical trauma, and ethnic skin. For example, skin diseases, such as acne, may leave dark spots after the condition clears. This type of hyperpigmentation is called post inflammatory hyperpigmentation. Post Inflammatory hyperpigmentation is the medical term given to the discoloration of the skin that follows an inflammatory wound. Post-inflammatory pigmentation develops when a wound, rash, pimple, or other stimuli causes skin inflammation, which triggers the skin to produce too much melanin. The excess melanin darkens and discolors the wounded area. This discoloration remains even after the wound or pimple has healed. The acne hyperpigmentation does not appear in all acne conditions. Mostly, it is common when people do "squeezing" and expose skin to direct sunlight right after. Damaged skin starts producing an abnormal amount of melanin and spots appear. It can take three to 24 months for post inflammatory pigmentation to fully fade, although, in some cases, it may take much longer and require treatment.

The esthetic industry offers several effective post inflammatory hyperpigmentation treatments. Most effective are chemical peels and microdermabrasion. The complete protocols of the chemical peel and microdermabrasion treatment are given in **Chapter 8: Microdermabrasion and Chemical Peels**. This chapter is also offering a detailed description of microdermabrasion procedure.

Before the actual treatment the esthetician should analyze the skin using Wood's lamp. A Wood's lamp is a device that emits ultraviolet (UV) light in the 365-nanometer range and it is commonly used by skin care experts to assist in the diagnosis of various pigment and infectious skin disorders. The Wood's lamp is must have tool to determine the location of melanin deposition, since melanin can be deposited in the epidermis or dermis.

Dermal hyperpigmentation is much more challenging to treat, while epidermal hyperpigmentation can be easily diminished with mild chemical peel. The examination has to be performed in a dark room by reviewing the affected area of the face under a Wood's lamp. When analyzing the skin under the Wood's lamp, an esthetician has to pay attention to the color of each pigment spot to determine how deep the pigmentation lays under the skin.

Tips for Observing Hyperpigmentation

Here are some helpful tips to keep in mind when observing hyperpigmentation:

- Increased melanin in the epidermis tends to be dark brown color.
- Melanin in the epidermis and high dermis is mostly brown with hints of gray or blue.

- Increased melanin in the dermis tends to be more grayish or blue.
- Mixed epidermal-dermal depositions are brown-gray.

More common cases of hyperpigmentation, like melasma and post inflammatory hyperpigmentation can be treated professionally at skin care salons, medi-spas, and dermatologist's office. Procedural treatments include various chemical peels and microdermabrasion. A series of treatments are usually needed to adequately fade the unwanted skin's pigmentation. Chemical peels provide almost immediate results for treating age spots for chloasma. In contrary, microdermabrasion slowly removes unwanted pigmentation over a series of treatments. 10 to 12 treatments are required to reach the desirable effect. I recommend that my signature Hyperpigmentation Facial include both microdermabrasion and a mild chemical peel, recommended in 10-12 sequential treatments, a week apart.

During the treatment, and particularly after, the results are reached wearing sunscreen is a must. The sunscreen must be "broad spectrum" (i.e. it blocks both UVA and UVB). A single day of excess sun without wearing sunscreen can undo months of treatment. I recommend at least SPF 60 if the client has undergone hyperpigmentation treatment and wants to protect the results.

Hyperpigmentation Facial Protocol

As I have mentioned above, my specific Hyperpigmentation Facial is characterized by the combination of light peel and microdermabrasion procedure in one session. This way, the client can see the improvement from the first treatment. However, only after 7 days, when skin peels off is improvement truly noticeable.

The microdermabrasion solution that I use to prepare skin for the microdermabrasion creates a slight peeling effect. But if you want to have stronger peel, you can add to the solution equal part of 10% salicylic acid. In severe cases of melasma, you can use straight 10% salicylic acid and alcohol solution. Apply the solution to the whole face and the neck right before the microdermabrasion. Wait for several minutes and allow the skin to calm down and follow with the procedure. If you want to reach a stronger peeling effect, the solution can be applied right after microdermabrasion, but this method cannot be used for sensitive skin.

For the formula of microdermabrasion solution, refer to the Step 4 of the treatment's protocol. Remember; tell your client that their skin is going to slightly peel for the following 5-7 days. On the second session of the microdermabrasion, the peel should be avoided. Instead just thoroughly and gently remove dead skin from the face with microdermabrasion tip. The third treatment should be performed as a first one, which will include the peel. And the following session there is no peel. Alternating these treatments, you will reach the best result by doing a total of 5 mild chemical peels and 10 microdermabrasion sessions without peel. The procedures should be done once per week.

- Step #1: Cleanse.

    Cleanse face with Gentle Cleansing Gel (Raya Lab, Inc) or any appropriate cleanser from your favorite skin care line. For the post inflammatory hyperpigmentation, I use a cleanser for problem skin as you do for acne treatment. Gentle Cleansing Gel is a great product, specially formulated for dry and sensitive skin, and it thoroughly cleans the skin, while slightly moisturizing with botanical extracts.

- Step #2: Exfoliate.

    After removing the cleanser with washcloth or sponges, perform exfoliation with an appropriate product. I like to use Enzyme Peeling Cream or Bamboo Facial Scrub manufactured by Raya Lab, Inc. The purpose of the scrub or enzyme peel is to remove dead cells from stratum corneum (first layer of epidermis) and softening the layer beneath. The Enzyme Peeling Cream is very effective as a non-abrasive scrub alternative for all skin types, including blemished and sensitive skin. It is based on aloe vera gel and contains fruit enzymes and botanical extracts.

    To remove the Enzyme Peeling Cream, gently roll off the mask with a tissue. If you are using the scrub type of exfoliator simply wash it with damp cellulose sponges or a washcloth.

- Step 3: Extract.

    Perform extraction if the skin is congested and plaqued with comedones. Steam the face for 10 min to open the pores and soften the black heads. Apply the extraction mask to help remove comedones without traumatizing the client's skin. My favorite extraction mask for normal and oily skin contains flaxseed meal. Simply mix one teaspoon of flaxseed meal with 3% H_2O_2 right before the steaming, and remove the mask with a wet towel right before the extraction. It is very important to disinfect the skin after the extraction, using an astringent or toner that has antibacterial properties. I use my Calendula tincture that I have mentioned before.

➤ Step #4: Apply microdermabrasion solution.

It is strongly recommended to perform microdermabrasion procedure on clean and de-oiled skin. In other words, skin has to contain no moisture or oils. Microdermabrasion solution is perfectly designed to prepare skin by removing all impurities and skin oil. Apply the microdermabrasion solution to the whole face and neck area and wait until it dries. Apply the solution a couple of times until the skin feels dry to the touch.

Microdermabrasion Solution Recipe

In a 6 oz glass container, add 3 oz of the Calendula tincture, 2 oz of Camphor spirits, and 1 oz of Witch hazel astringent. Mix well and store in dark place. Camphor spirits can be easily found at drugstore.

➤ Step #5: Perform microdermabrasion procedure.

Perform the microdermabrasion procedure on the whole face and neck, according to the skin lines, especially concentrating on pigment spots. Sometimes, redness may occur when you reach the dermal layer of the skin. It is quite normal since deep microdermabrasion reaches the dermal layer of the skin, where blood vessels are located. It is proven that deep abrasion provides faster skin rejuvenation, since the skin tries to "heal" itself by rapid production of new cells.

➤ Step #6: Apply a Vitamin C serum.

Here I want to emphasize the importance of post-microdermabrasion treatment. To my knowledge, most microdermabrasion treatments are limited to abrasion procedure with a following application of the moisturizer or serum. That microdermabrasion lasts about 30 min and is known as a "lunch time" treatment. Personally, I think it is not an effective treatment because microdermabrasion itself just deeply exfoliates the skin, but it is extremely important what the treatment is that you provide right after.

The effect of microdermabrasion is to stimulate new cells production by removing upper layers of epidermis. The natural skin's protecting mechanism will start produce new cells. Therefore, it is important to apply the best ingredients to help the body manufacture new healthy cells. For example, Vitamin C is one of the most important vitamins for anti-aging treatments, since it is used by the dermis to manufacture collagen. Our body's mechanisms limit the amount of Vitamin

C to be available for our skin. Using a Vitamin C serum to be applied topically is the way to directly protect and rejuvenate the skin.

Therefore, the next step of the treatment includes a Vitamin C serum application, anti-aging massage, and bleaching mask application.

> Step #7: Provide a lympho-drainage and healing massage.

A lympho-drainage massage will be greatly beneficial for aging skin. It promotes toxin removal, increases blood flow, and speeds up healing the processes of the skin. For detailed facial massage techniques, refer to the **Chapter 6: Skin Aging.**

For post inflammatory pigmentation treatment, include 5 min of healing massage, using the same technique as for an Acne Facial. Follow with bleaching mask application for 15- 20 min. Remove mask with damp washcloth and finish with bleaching cream.

Hyperpigmentation Masks

Below are a few formulas that can help to illuminate unwanted pigmentation and post- inflammatory spots.

Recipes to diminish large pores

Mask with egg whites and 10% solution of hydrogen peroxide.

10% or 35% solutions of food grade hydrogen peroxide (H2O2) can be found in health food stores or vitamin stores. Mix one part of 35% H2O2 with two parts of distilled water to receive 10% H2O2. Mix beaten egg whites with a few drops of 10% solution of H2O2 and spread carefully over the pigment spots. Eyes should be covered with a cotton pad.

Remove dried out mask with wet sponges. The mask helps to shrink enlarged pores and lighten up unwanted pigmentation.

Mask with Egg Whites and Alum Powder

Add to one beaten egg white, 1/4-teaspoon alum powder. Mix thoroughly and apply on the face until it dries. Remove with wet sponges. If dry mask is hard to remove, use a wet towel to soften the mask.

You can add to the mixture fresh squeezed lemon juice to reach stronger bleaching effect.

<u>*Mask for Oily Skin with 3% Hydrogen Peroxide and Citric Acid*</u>

Kaolin 1 oz (30gr)
Citric acid 1/4 teaspoon
3%H2O2 1oz (30 g)

<u>*Bleaching Mask for Dry and Sun Damaged Skin*</u>

Mix one teaspoon of sour cream and one teaspoon of fresh squeezed lemon juice. Add a few drops of 35% H2O2. Apply on the skin for 40 min.

Home routine between the sessions require daily application of the bleaching cream for night time and application of sunscreen for the day. Multiple topical modalities are known to diminish skin's dark pigment spots.

Hydroquinone is a widely used treatment for hyperpigmentation. Hydroquinone works by blocking the enzyme responsible for melanin production, thereby lightening the skin. Hydroquinone creams often contain additional lightening ingredients, such as kojic acid, glycolic acid, tretinoin, and other retinoids, or Vitamin C. These combination creams can give better results than using hydroquinone alone.

It is available over-the-counter at 1% or 2% strength. However, the lower percentage creams usually are not as effective as lotions with higher concentration of hydroquinone. The creams that contain 4% and 6% of hydroquinone are available by prescription only. However, high percentages of hydroquinone can cause severe irritation for sensitive skin. There is a bleaching cream that has great bleaching effect that I prefer over hydroquinone, and it does not cause irritation. I have been using this product for years to diminish melasma and post inflammatory blemishes. The cream contains 35% food grade hydrogen peroxide and can easily be prepared, finding all the necessarily ingredients in health food stores.

<u>*H2O2 (Hydrogen Peroxide) cream for Nighttime*</u>

35% Hydrogen Peroxide 1 oz (30 g)
Vaseline 5 oz (150 g)
Lanolin oil 5oz (150 g)
Water distill 3oz (100gr)

Mix lanolin with distilled water until fully absorbed. Then add Vaseline to reach smooth texture. Lastly, add 35% H_2O_2 constantly mixing. Mix until all H_2O_2 is completely absorbed by lanolin-water base.

The cream has to be stored in a cool place and placed in a large glass container, since it will double in volume. The cream can be used for hyperpigmentation treatments as a facial mask for 15-20 minutes. Also, it can be used daily, applying it directly on pigment spots as an overnight treatment.

<u>Bleaching Cream with Camphor</u>

Camphor cream designed for dull, congested skin to diminish post-inflammatory pigment spots.
Camphor crystals 2/3 oz (20 g)
Salicylic acid powder 1/3 oz (10gr)
Zinc Oxide ointment 3 oz (90gr)
Vaseline 3 oz (90gr)
Camphor crystals and salicylic acid powder dilute in 1 oz of 96% grain alcohol ("Ever clear") until all crystals are gone. Then slowly mix it with zinc oxide ointment and Vaseline. Store it in glass container, and use it as a mask to bleach post acne pigment blemishes.

<u>Lemon Cream to Reduce Unwanted Pigmentation</u>

35% Hydrogen Peroxide 1 oz (30gr)
Citric acid 1 teaspoon (5gr)
Lanolin 1 tablespoon 0, 5 oz. (15gr)
Distill water 1oz (30g)
Zinc oxide ointment 10% 8 oz (240gr)
Mix citric acid with water and slowly with lanolin to absorb mixture. Then add zinc oxide ointment, and at the end, gradually add 35% H_2O_2 until it is all absorbed by the ointment. Store the cream in a large container, since it will double in volume. The cream can be used to diminish unwanted hyperpigmentation if used on daily basis. Besides, it can be used for salon treatments as a bleaching product, especially if it is used along with Galvanic method.

Galvanic Method

Galvanic method is an excellent tool to treat hyperpigmentation of the skin, and it refers to skin treatment that enhances the absorption of nutrients by bringing the nourishing products deep into skin using the anode (+) and the cathode (-) of electric current. The Galvanic method can assist in reducing hyperpigmentation, anti-aging treatment, acne treatment, etc. The benefits of this method refer to the painless and precise application of the cosmetic products in order to achieve the maximum penetration on treated area. Therefore, the Galvanic procedure can give deeper penetration of any cosmetic ingredients in comparison with regular topical application.

The substance used for the treatment should have the ability to disassociate ions (electrolytes). The device has two electrodes; one metal roll-on that applies directly to the skin and an opposite polarity electrode that the client holds in their hand. For better conductivity of the electric current, the opposite electrode has to be wrapped with gauze that has been saturated in a water-salt solution. Meanwhile, the metal roll-on electrode has to be wrapped with gauze that has been saturated with a cosmetic product.

Before the treatment, it is important to know the polarity of the cosmetic substance. For example, for hyperpigmentation treatment, I use a higher percentage of hydrogen peroxide (5% or 10%). The H2O2 is negative and the machine has to be on (-). Duration of the application is about 15 min.

Vitamin C solution (2% -5%) and aloe vera gel have a negative charge as well. I use these products for anti-aging Galvanic treatments. In addition, ionophores, with ichthammol ointment, give excellent results to eliminate inflammation and heal the skin, and they can be used to treat cystic acne. Electrophores (ionophores) with 2% hydrocortisone ointment can be used to treat dermatitis. There are varieties of anti-aging skin care serums manufactured by professional cosmetic companies that have been utilized for Galvanic treatments; most of them contain Vitamin C and hyaluronic acid.

Chapter 8: Microdermabrasion & Chemical Peels

Microdermabrasion is a cosmetic procedure in which the stratum corneum (upper layer of the human skin) is partially or completely removed by light abrasion. It is one of the three most commonly performed dermatology treatments in the United States, and its relatively low cost makes it a practical choice for patients with minor skin problems and early signs of aging.

From minimizing fine lines to diminishing skin pores, microdermabrasion provides many benefits. Microdermabrasion sloughs off the dead and dull surface layers of the skin, stimulating an increase in collagen production and rejuvenation. Many patients see dramatic improvements in the tone, texture, and color of treated areas after just one treatment.

Microdermabrasion can also improve:

1. Mild scaring,
2. Unwanted pigmentation,
3. Fine lines,
4. Skin pores texture, and
5. Oily and congested skin.

Different methods include mechanical abrasion from jets with aluminum oxide crystals, fine organic particles, or diamond tip. When microdermabrasion procedure first became popular over 20 years ago, the majority of microdermabrasion equipment used aluminum oxide or baking soda crystals to provide abrasion action. Crystal-free microdermabrasion (diamond tip is used for abrasive purposes) became popular in recent years, due to some obvious advantages over crystal equipment.

Diamond Tip vs. Crystal Tip

Here are few good reasons why diamond tip devices are superior to crystal tip.

Firstly, diamond is actually four times harder than corundum (aluminum oxide) crystals. Secondly, the diamond tips are reusable and last for long time versus aluminum oxide crystals, which have to be disposed of after each treatment and continuously refilled. Next crystal-free tips are easier to use and unlikely to leave tiny particles in the eyes, nose, and mouth. Besides, it has been an ongoing controversy related to safety of aluminum oxide crystals, since it can possibly contribute to an accumulation of aluminum in the human body.

I work with both types of machines, and they both give good results, but I prefer to use the diamond tip machine for the reasons mentioned above.

Microdermabrasion does not present any serious risks when performed by a qualified esthetician. Some side effects may include slight skin irritation in the form of redness and increased skin sensitivity. In the previous chapter of the book, I have described all the details of the Hyperpigmentation Facial and included a step-by-step microdermabrasion treatment protocol. I am expecting that skin professionals who read my book have already received decent microdermabrasion training and have a pretty good idea of how to operate microdermabrasion equipment.

Chemical Peels

Chemical peel is one of the oldest cosmetic procedures in the world, and it was performed in ancient Egypt, Greece, and Rome to help people achieve smoother, more beautiful skin.

A chemical peel is a caustic procedure that burns the outer layers of the skin, revealing a younger, fresher looking skin. A chemical peel can be performed by various agents including "fruit acids" (glycolic, alpha-hydroxy, or lactic acid), trichloroacetic acid (TCA), salicylic acid (Beta-hydroxy), phenol, and other chemicals.

Light chemical peels, like a glycolic peel, do not require much downtime, and the skin recovers very fast. You can see immediate skin improvement. With deep peels, like TCA, 20% salicylic acid, recovery time can be up to two weeks.

TCA peel (trichloroacetic acid) is one time application and does not require layering or taping; methods are used with salicylic acid peels.

A chemical peel can restore a more youthful appearance to wrinkled, unevenly pigmented, sun-damaged, or blotchy skin.

Benefits of a chemical peel procedure include:

- Visible improvement of the skin's texture
- Significant reduction of unwanted facial pigmentation, freckles, age spots, and chloasma
- Diminishing of fine lines on the lip and forehead area
- Reduction of appearance of stretch marks, scars, and post acne blemishes
- Significant improvement of acne conditions

Chemical peel is not recommended for people with the following skin conditions:

- Kelloid or hypertrophic scars (thick scars)
- Past and acute herpes lesions
- Allergy on the chemical agent
- Wart on the face and neck
- Recent radiation treatment for cancer
- Recent usage of Acutance or Retin-A
- Recent microdermabrasion completed sessions
- Recent laser resurfacing procedure
- Sunburn or significant sun exposure in the last week

All chemical peels involve applying a chemical solution to remove the outer layers of skin so that a smoother, more evenly pigmented, glowing layer of skin can appear. There are three basic categories of chemical peels. Each type works differently, and produces different results. It is recommended to successfully complete a patch test to the area of skin you intend to treat. This consists of applying the peeling solution to the small part of the skin near the area you plan to treat. If the skin responds without any allergic reaction, you can proceed with the peeling treatment for the entire area.

To perform chemical peels, the esthetician has to have extensive training and some experience. Many skin care specialists, even after training, do not know how human skin will react to certain chemical agents. For those who want to learn how to properly perform chemical peels, I want to present the five most common treatments in detail. If you follow these steps, and my personal suggestions, your success is guaranteed.

Common Chemical Peel Treatments

Skin peels are conducted by applying professional strength solutions of glycolic (35-45%), lactic, or salicylic acid (10%). They burn off only the outer layers of the skin to smooth out fine wrinkles and rough, dry skin. Peels may also be used to improve the texture of sun-damaged skin, balance out skin pigmentation, or diminish post inflammatory acne scars. These peels are often repeated to achieve the desired results. Six to ten sessions, each a week apart, are recommended.

❖ **Glycolic Peel**

Glycolic acid is generally regarded to be the most active and beneficial of the Alpha-Hydroxy-Acids (AHA) in skin care. Glycolic acid is a superficial peeling agent that is made from sugar cane. It effectively exfoliates the skin, reduces fine lines, and helps to lighten hyperpigmentation. Once applied, glycolic acid reacts with the outer layer of skin (epidermal) cells, weakening the binding properties of the lipids (the "glue") that hold the dead cells together. This is the mechanism that allows the damaged outer skin layer to "peel" off to reveal the underlying new skin cells, thus giving skin an even, untarnished texture. In addition, glycolic acid can penetrate into the new skin cell's membrane; stimulating them to generate collagen and elastic fibers that overall improves skin's condition.

The peel may be beneficial for the following skin problems:

- Superficial wrinkles of the face, neck, upper chest, arms,
- Uneven pigmentation problems
- Enlarged facial pores
- Post-inflammatory acne scars
- Age spots
- Sun-damaged skin

The application of glycolic or 10% salicylic acid is relatively fast and simple. There will not be noticeable peeling, just a sloughing action that will leave skin feeling smooth and looking refreshed. The dry, congested surface sebum that makes skin dull and clogs pores will be dissolves and removed. Other cosmetic treatment programs, such as microdermabrasion, electrolysis, depilatories, waxing, bleaching agents, exfoliating products, like Retin- A, should be discontinued one week immediately before the peeling procedure.

During a chemical peel, most clients experience a warm to hot sensation that may last about 5 to 10 minutes and may be followed by some stinging. Depending upon the type of peel applied, there may be a mild to severe sunburn-like sensation, but this mostly refers to medium and deep chemical peels. The gentlest type of peel, a superficial peel, usually produces redness, which is followed by scaling that lasts three to five days.

I use professional strength of glycolic acid (35-45%) called Glycolic Bio-rectifying exfoliator, manufactured by Raya Lab, Inc., and this product is available only for licensed professionals.

➢ Step #1: Cleanse.

Clean the face with appropriate cleanser, using cleanser application technique. Wash away facial cleanser with damp sponges or washcloth.

➢ Step #2: Exfoliate.

Use this exfoliation step only for dry and aging skin. For oily and blemished skin, exfoliation with a facial scrub is not recommended.

The purpose or the exfoliation to remove dead cells from the outer layer of epidermis for better glycolic acid penetration

Remove scrub with damp cello sponges or a damp washcloth.

➢ Step #3: Apply glycolic acid.

On smooth clean skin, apply glycolic acid, using a large cotton swab, following the skin lines. Begin with the forehead down to the base of the neck. Keep the product on the skin for 5 min, and slough it off using a soft tissue. The product will roll off from the skin along with the layers of dead cells of the epidermis.

Follow with the same step, two more times, for a total of three applications. Each time, keep glycolic acid on for 5 min. The client may experience a slight stinging of the face along with mild redness. That is normal reaction of the skin on any peeling agent from normal to sensitive types. Needless to say, that you have to pay extra attention when you treat sensitive skin. Test the small part of skin on the back of the hand to see how skin will react to the product.

➢ Step #4: Apply the nourishing mask.

After the last application, remove the rest of glycolic acid with a damp washcloth and follow with the nourishing mask. For dry and mature skin, the mask has to be creamy with rejuvenating properties. For oily and skin with acne, use an antibacterial facial mask. To finish the treatment, apply a moisturizer that is appropriate to skin type.

❖ **10% Salicylic Peel**

To perform this treatment, you have to use 10% salicylic acid solution. You can purchase it from professional skin care companies, or you can simply prepare it yourself.

There are many websites that sell salicylic acid powder. All you have to do just Google "salicylic acid powder" and you will see several companies that are selling this product. Usually, it runs up to $35.00 for 4 ounces. The substance dissolves only in 95% food grain alcohol, known as Everclear. It is a brand of neutral grain spirit, available in concentrations of 75.5% alcohol (151 proof) and 95% alcohol (190 proof).

To obtain 100mg of 10% solution of salicylic acid, slowly add 10 g of salicylic acid powder to 100ml of Everclear (95%). Store the mixture in dark glass container, and keep it in a cool, dark place.

You can also purchase ready-to use solution from this website that sells 2 ounce of 10% salicylic peel: http://www.naturalskinshop.net/product_p/prxs10p.htm or http://perfect-peel-solutions-llc.amazonwebstore.com.

"Perfect-peel-solutions, LLC" sells varieties of mild and deep chemical peel solutions at very reasonable prices. On this website, you can purchase 10% salicylic acid peel, 20% salicylic peel, Jessner's solution, TCA, and much more.

➢ Step #1: Cleanse.

Start with the facial cleanser appropriate for certain skin type. Remove it with damp cello sponges.

➢ Step #2: Exfoliate.

Proceed with a mild scrub to exfoliate dead cells from the stratum corneum (upper epidermal layer). You can use any facial scrub from your professional skin care line, or you can try Bamboo scrub from Raya Lab, Inc. This herbal based exfoliating cream combines finely ground bamboo with jojoba beads and micro-fine French talc. It effectively removes dead cells of epidermis, lifts away dull, dry skin to improve texture and healthy clarity. Remember; do not perform any exfoliation for skin with acne lesions and inflamed pustules.

> Step #3: Apply salicylic acid.

Prepare skin for the salicylic acid peel after removing scrub with damp cellulose sponges. Apply Calendula lotion to disinfect the skin and remove residue of oils and moisture.

Next, saturate a large cotton swab in the 10% salicylic acid solution and apply with even strokes for entire face, starting with forehead. The client will be experiencing a strong burning sensation and slight redness may appear. Wait until the burning sensation stops, and apply the solution one more time. Usually, it is enough for two applications to reach the desirable effect, but in case of thick and extremely oily skin, you may add one more application.

> Step #4: Apply aloe vera gel and effleurage.

To reduce the redness and calm the skin, use aloe vera gel, spreading it on the entire face with light effleurage.

> Step #5: Apply a calming mask.

Final step concludes with a calming mask application. The mask has to contain aloe vera, kaolin, and allantoin. If you cannot find a mask with this ingredient in your skin care line, you can prepare it yourself.

Calming Mask Recipe

Aloe Vera gel 1oz (30 ml)
Kaolin, 1 oz (30 g)
Allantoin 1 teaspoon (5gr)
Calendula tincture 1 tablespoon (15 g)

Leave the mask on for 15-20 min and remove with damp cello sponges. Follow with an appropriate moisturizer.

Raya Lab, Inc. has professional skin care products that have been dedicated to supporting skin care professionals toward creating varieties of cosmetics suitable for all skin treatment and skin needs. Cucumber Ice Sorbet Masque is a very gentle facial cooling gel. It is recommended as a calming and soothing regimen for all skin types, including sensitive skin. A natural synergy of herbal extracts (cucumber, chamomile and aloe vera) provides an anti-irritant effect and helps to reduce redness and inflammation associated with in-salon skin chemical peels. Disinfecting and Bleaching Powder Masque contains kaolin, zinc oxide, boric acid and powdered aloe vera that can be successfully used as a post chemical peel treatment.

Aloe Vera and Herbs Soothing Gel is an effective soothing, moisturizing, and skin-conditioning product made from natural aloe vera and botanical extracts. This gel comforts red and irritated skin and can be used right after chemical agent application.

- **Seaweed (Spongilla) Peel**

Seaweed (spongilla) is a unique product that I have been using in my practice for years. I named the facial treatment "Seaweed Peel", and it can be used as anti-aging treatment and for acne treatments as well. Spongilla was commonly used in Russia and Ukraine to treat joints inflammation and skin disorders. It has unique ability to "digest" the top layers of epidermis to provide younger looking skin. It is also widely used for post inflammatory acne scars, since it is effectively reduces visibility of acne blemishes and post acne pigment spots.

To prepare the mixture for seaweed peel, the powdered spongilla (it comes in powder form) should be combined with 3% hydrogen peroxide. Apply the mixture on the clients face for 15 min and remove it with damp washcloth, gently sloughing off the mask. Then wash the entire face with wet cello sponge, and apply a moisturizer suitable for particular skin type.

Immediately following post application, a healthy appearing glow becomes evident due to the enhanced blood circulation in the treated skin. Speckles penetrated through epidermis communicate their presence and effectiveness via a unique tingling sensation to the touch. The erythematic and tingling sensation of the skin gradually fades over the following 12-24 hours. This product is truly unique and completely safe for all types of skin. However, I will not recommend it for rosacea skin conditions as well as for extremely sensitive skin.

To my knowledge, some websites sell the spongilla by itself or products that include it. Do your search, and it can make an exceptional addition to your services. I guarantee that not many estheticians are aware of the exceptional quality of spongilla, and it can become an exclusive treatment.

- **Jessner's Peel**

Jessner's peel is considered to be a mild peel, but it achieves better results than Alpha Hydroxy Acid peels and can be appropriate for clients whose skin requires a deeper peeling. Jessner's peel can be very beneficial to lighten areas of hyperpigmentation as well as to improve sun-damaged skin. In addition, *Jessner's peel* has been used to illuminate mild acne and acne scars. Jessner's solution causes the top layers of skin to flake off, while also stimulating the deeper layers of skin. The dermis stimulated by the Jessner's solution will produce new fibroblasts and collagen fibers, causing the reduction of the depth of lines and wrinkles. Repetitive peeling will improve tone, texture, and quality of the skin.

Jessner's solution contains 14% salicylic acid, 14% lactic acid, and 14% resorcinol, combined and formed into one amazing solution, specifically designed for skin resurfacing, Results of this light-to-medium depth peel are fantastic with the combination of these 3 very unique chemical peel agents.

Lactic acid is great for people with sensitive skin or for those who are unable to withstand the glycolic acid peels. This acid is also well known for its ability to kill germs, toxins, and shed dead cells, as well as maintain the pH level of the skin. This regulating is crucial for keeping the skin healthy, free of dirt, oil, and germs, and to provide an overall smooth, even texture.

Resorcinol is great for a variety of skin conditions that include acne, warts, calluses, dull rough skin, eczema, corns, psoriasis, and many others. Resorcinol helps to clear up the skin of blemishes and prevent infection, which allows for faster healing and recovery periods.

Salicylic acid is a perfect remedy for those who suffer from extremely oily skin, severe acne (acne vulgaris), clogged pores, and blackheads. Salicylic acid is an excellent deep pore cleanser with many anti-aging properties.

You can purchase Jessner's solution online or from skin care companies that provide educational classes on chemical peel. Here is a website address for the company, where I am buying my supplies for the skin peels: www.perfect-peel-solutions-llc.amazonwebstore.com

Treatment protocol for Jessner's peel is the same as 10% salicylic peel. Please, refer to the description above.

- ❖ **TCA (Trichloroacetic Acid) Peel**

This is an effective mild-to-deep peeling agent. The higher percentage (35% +) of TCA is considered as deep chemical peel and can be performed only by dermatologist. 10-15% and 20% TCA peel can be done by an experienced esthetician that completed appropriate training in chemical skin peels. Chemical peel with 20% TCA is an option for people with severe melasma that is unresponsive to topical bleaching agents. TCA peel is also ideally suited for people who have undergone other peel treatments and now require a deeper peel for more effective results.

TCA actively treats surface wrinkles, superficial blemishes, and unwanted pigmentation. In contrary to the salicylic peel that mostly is used for the face, TCA can be used for face, neck, and hands.

TCA Peel Protocol

- Step #1: Cleanse.

    Apply a facial cleanser on the client's skin and remove it with damp washcloth or wet cello sponges.

- Step #2: Exfoliate.

    Application of mild scrub or enzymatic exfoliator is required. You can also use one application of 10% AHA or glycolic acid. The exfoliator will remove the top layer of the epidermis and prepare skin for deeper exfoliation.

- Step #3: Apply TCA solution.

    To apply the TCA solution, saturate a large cotton swab with 1 ml of the solution. Apply the TCA to the entire face evenly starting with the forehead. Follow the skin lines, avoiding eyes and eye area. For the anti-aging treatment, apply solution on the neck as well, starting from the jaw towards the clavicle bone. The client will experience a strong burning sensation. You may need use a fan or cold-water compress to relieve the uncomfortable sensation.

    For the initial application, leave the solution on for 30 sec. During this time, the skin may frost and turn white, depending on the concentration and number of applications. This is normal, and the frost will disappear within 30 minutes.

    The change in coloration of the skin to a whitish tint is called frost. This represents the end of stage of the chemical peel and shows that keratin agglutination has occurred.

    Proceed with a second application for deeper peel. Second application can be a little longer, for up to 1 min. For initial TCA peel, leave the solution for 1-2 minutes maximum. As tolerance to the peel increases, the peel solution may be left on for longer periods, but never for more than 10 min. Do not repeat it more than three times.

- Step #4: Neutralize.

    Neutralization of the chemical peeling agent is an important step once the esthetician has achieved the proper depth of the peel, which is determined either by the frost or how much time the application lasted.

Neutralization can be achieved with cold water or a wet, cool towel applied to the face. Therefore, wash the face with the cold water and sponge to remove the residue of the solution and follow with application of Aloe Vera to relieve the irritation.

> Step #5: Apply a calming mask.

Proceed with the calming mask application to calm the redness and relieve burning. Gently remove mask with the wet cello sponges or damp washcloth. Follow with rich moisturizer to relieve tightness.

It is important to give your client recommendations on how to take care of their skin during the recovery period. Within a few days, the skin will tighten and darken- and then begin to crack a peel for the next four to seven days. At this point, the smoother, youthful-looking layer of skin will emerge. Moisturizing is very important after the skin has start peel off, and harsh abrasive agents should be avoided. The client has to protect their skin with a good sunblock and avoid direct sunlight and tanning beds.

❖ **Jessner's + TCA Peel**

This is a popular combination of two peeling solutions that can provide an effective medium depth peel and produce an outstanding level of controlled skin peel without the risk of side effects. Why is it so beneficial to use a combination peel? The Jessner's solution was found effective in destroying the epidermal barrier by breaking up individual epidermal cells. This process allows a deeper penetration of the TCA and more even application of the peeling solution. If Jessner's solution is applied first to the skin and then followed with mild form of TCA, the deeper results will be without the risks associated with deeper chemical peels.

To perform these peels, follow the same steps of the previous protocol. But, before using 20% TCA, apply the Jessner's solution to the area to be treated. In other words, after about 1-2 minutes of Jessner's application, follow with application of TCA over the same area. The skin will frost with TCA but will diminish after 30 minutes. Do not leave TCA on the skin more that 3 min. After the application, wash it off with damp washcloth or wet cello sponges and follow with calming mask and appropriate moisturizer. I recommend using Azulen Soothing Masque manufactured by Raya Lab, Inc. This unscented, light emollient formula is and effective addition to any skin peel procedure. It provides instant moisture relief with long lasting soothing and comfort effects.

❖ Phenol Acid Peel

One of the most common deep chemical peels is the Phenol Acid peel. Phenol acid is the strongest chemical peel solution, and it is used for the deepest possible chemical peel. Phenol peel is usually performed only in dermatologist office, since small sedation or anesthesia is required. Phenol peels are used to treat skin with coarse wrinkles and blotchiness. They may also be effectively used to treat patients with pre-cancerous growths.

Phenol peels should be used with caution, because they can cause permanent lightening of the skin. For this reason, phenol peels are not recommended for most people with very dark skin tones.

Full-face phenol peels take approximately one to two hours, but small-area phenol peels (such as on the upper lip) may take about 10-15 minutes. Unlike AHA and TCA peels, phenol peels are only used once to create dramatic results.

❖ 20% Salicylic Acid Peel

The other well-known deep chemical peel is the 20% salicylic acid peel. Salicylic acid, a Beta-Hydroxy Acid, is a highly effective, superficial peeling agent, and it is one of the most effective ingredients to combat the cause of excessive facial oil, acne, and blemishes. It also provides excellent rejuvenating results. Salicylic acid loosens and removes aging cells, oil, and debris attached to skin's surface.

The 20% salicylic peel is considered deep to medium peel and can be performed by an esthetician that has an experience in chemical peels.

I am referring you to my signature treatment with 20% of salicylic acid, and if you follow all steps properly, it can produce outstanding results. The fine lines become less visible and unwanted pigmentation can be removed by 90%. You can use the peel for the purposes of improving acne scars, chicken pox scars, and post pregnancy melasma.

The downside of this peel is the fact that clients have to avoid any moisture on the face for 7 days. Taking showers has to be carefully done, avoiding getting water on the face, especially during first days of treatment. The whole peeling procedure includes five sequential 20% salicylic acid applications. Therefore, in this type of facial peel, five consecutive sessions are needed to complete the process. Every session will take no more than 30 minutes total. 20% salicylic solution can be purchased from professional skin care companies or from the mentioned above website.

Day 1

After face cleansing with appropriate facial cleanser, wipe the whole face with 2% salicylic acid solution (2% salicylic spirits) and follow with five 20% Salicylic acid applications in following sequence. First, apply the solution on both sides of the cheeks, then on the chin, nose, and the forehead. Avoid the eyes area and lips. For better protection around eye area and lips, use a small amount of any moisturizer. The skin will turn red after initial application of salicylic acid solution, and the client will experience a strong burning sensation. Use a fan to provide relief from burning and stinging. After the second application, skin can turn white and frosty. To neutralize the frost, use 2% Salicylic acid solution until it all gone and skin returns to normal.

Perform five applications in total; each time removing the frost from the skin with 2% salicylic spirit. Do not apply any moisture afterward, and advise your clients to not wash their face at all. Water and any moisturizers should be avoided during this peel. In contrary, medicated powder or baby powder should be used to keep the face dry.

Day 2

This session includes a total of ten applications of 20% salicylic acid. Perform 10 applications of 20% salicylic acid solution in the same manner as described above.

Day 3 and Day 4

Both of these days, perform only six applications of 20% salicylic acid; each time, remove the frosty film with 2% salicylic spirit.

Day 5

On the last day of treatment, apply the 20% salicylic solution 5 times.

Day 6

After done with all sessions, you should advise the client not to use any moisture or water on the face. Instead, to keep the skin dry, they must use baby powder. This will help to speed up the skin peeling process and old skin layers rejection.

Day 7

By this day the client's face will feel very tight, covered with light brown crust of old skin and possibly start peeling in some places. To remove the crust, you need to steam the client's face (10- 15 min) and gently remove pieces of dead skin. Do not force the skin to be removed unless it is really loose. Forcefully peeling the skin may create scarring. Instead, use petroleum jelly or lanolin cream on the new skin. By day 8 and 9 all "dead" skin should peel off and smooth, youthful looking skin will appears. The client should be instructed to use good moisturizer and stay out of the sun.

In conclusion, I want to mention the dangers related to performing chemical peels by inexperienced persons. Improperly done peeling procedures can lead to serious complications, including scarring, infection, swelling, change in skin tone, and cold sore outbreaks. Skin reactions to the chemical ingredients included in peels can vary among individuals. If you are just starting practicing chemical peels, it is important to start with light peels and always perform a patch testing in a small area of the skin.

Chapter 9:
Skin Care for Male Clients

When I was working as a dermatologist in Ukraine, the percentage of male clients were about 30% of all my clients. Most of them were teenagers or young men who had moderate to severe acne skin conditions. It is a fact that puberty brings much more acne problems to men than women of the same age. It is related to elevated testosterone production when male teenagers start reaching puberty stage. Besides, young men, it seems do not care for their skin as much as girls do, and only when problems gets worse do they start seeking professional help.

As I mentioned above, the people in my country, when they have skin problems, think of estheticians first, rather than doctors. Because well-trained beauticians know how to deal with acne problems and offer many varieties of procedures to combat skin disorders.

Since I began my practice in the United States, the percentage of male clients dropped dramatically. Once in a while, the gentlemen who want a deep pore cleaning will sign up for the appointment. But, as far as teenage acne problems, all of them prefer to visit a dermatologist instead. That was a proof for my assumption that the reputation of domestic estheticians was not strong enough for people to expect have a success with acne problems.

Men skin care products were limited to aftershave lotions and some hair product. Facial products were mostly privileged for women. Strangely enough, a common bias says that men skin care products and routines do not exist and that these beauty procedures are only meant for women. Of course, it is absolute nonsense, since men's skin requires skin care just as much as women do.

Skin care for men began picking up in the last 10 years, and now actually there are many stores that exclusively sell male skin care products. According to statistics, men have become more interested in skin care cosmetics, and a higher demand for male skin care products has drastically increased in the past 20 years. Men like hair and skin care products specifically designed for the male population since the structure of their hair and the skin are somewhat different than women. For instance, male hair is usually oilier, due to an abundance of androgens (male reproductive hormone).

The structure of skin also has specific differences. The epidermis of their skin is twice as thick as female skin for the reason of the presence of androgens and regular shaving. In addition, the quantity of melanin cells in the epidermal layer of male skin is much larger than in women's skin. The sebaceous glands are bigger and produce more oil. Therefore, their skin is more protected from sun damage and other environmental factors that greatly contribute to the fact that male skin ages slower. Based on those facts, cosmetic companies are beginning to manufacture skin care products that are only suitable to men's skin.

Raya Lab, Inc. is able to develop many excellent skin care products for oily and problem skin. Camphor Soufflé or Blemish Control Gel are excellent cleansers for oily and comedonic men's skin. Blemish Control astringent is highly effective, and recommended only for very oily and blemished skin types. It contains Vitamin B complex that helps normalize the pH balance of the skin and regulate oil gland secretion. Bio-Drying Lotion is an effective acne control lotion that dries up blemishes, reduces tissue redness, and lessens irritation. Vitamin B Day Cream is a daily moisturizer for problem skin and complements this entire product line to help with the problem skin. This company also manufactures varieties of professional products for salons that increase estheticians' chances to successfully combat acne skin disorders.

In addition, as a skin care professionals, you have to educate your male clients on the importance of salon treatments along with home treatments. When I first opened my skin care business, I even conducted a small educational seminar for men who work at the banks, real estate agencies, and other establishments, where male employees were prevailing. Indeed, it helped me to build my male clientele rapidly, and it also helped men to recognize the importance of skin care routines. For many of them, a personal consultation with skin-expert was a discovery that skin care is not just a "women" thing; it is a necessity for any human.

During the initial consultation with your male client, you should be able to identify their concerns and choose the right product according to their skin type. To choose what is the best skin care routine for your male client, you need consider his age, his type of skin (oily, comedonic, dry), and any existing skin problems (acne, rosacea, keratosis, warts, sensitivity to any products, etc).

First Type: "Normal"

If the pores are small and unclogged and have very few blemishes, we can say that it is within the "normal" type. This type of skin does not shine after washing, and it is rosy and elastic. If the man is still under 30 years old, it should be enough to do two steps of skin care routine during the day: cleansing and moisturizing.

The majority of men still are using commercial hand soaps to wash their face. Your duty as an esthetician is to tell them the truth about the soap, regardless of whether it is handmade or commercial. Bar soap strips the skin's natural oils and is strongly alkaline, weakening the skin's protective acid mantle. Soap also leaves an invisible residue behind, dulling the skin's surface. In other words, there is nothing worse than regular, old-fashioned soap. Instead, you should recommend the use of a facial cleanser.

Over the course of a day, a man's face collects oil in an area known as the T-zone (across the forehead and down the nose). The facial cleanser is a pH-balanced product that effectively removes skin impurities without drying and irritation. Water-based protective moisturizer has be a key part of the daily skin care. Cleansing and moisturizing the skin has to be done twice per day: morning and night.

Second Type: "Oily"

Frequent blemishes, black and white heads, clogged pores, especially in the nose area and upper cheeks, determine an oily type. A man's skin type can also be recognized as oily if it appears to shine after washing the face, and it is extremely smooth without fine lines and wrinkles. A special type of man skin care product is needed to improve this skin's condition. Products for oily and problem skin are recommended.

Washing the face with the pH-balanced cleanser has to be done twice per day in the morning and at night. Proper facial cleanser will help to minimize oily build-up without over drying your skin. While a cleanser can wash away the oily sheen, an astringent or toner is the essential preventative tool. Blemish control lotion or astringent has to be added after cleansing, following with water-based moisturizer. A series of facial treatments by skin care professionals can be extremely helpful to improve skin condition.

Third Type: "Dry"

Dry skin is identified if pores are difficult to see or if pores are small. Wrinkles and fine lines, the appearance of crow's feet and flaky, thin, or transparent epidermis layers are also signs of dry skin. This problem appears mostly to men over 40 years old; therefore, anti-aging skin products have to be considered as a daily skin care routine. Anti-aging skin care products usually target this problem as many males do suffer from a lack of moisture.

Morning care should include an exfoliating cleanser to slough off the dead epidermal layer. Additionally, an exfoliating scrub should be used once or twice per week. Toner can bring skin pH balance to normal, and a good moisturizer will protect skin from over-drying.

The use of a cream around eyes is just as important as moisturizing the face. There are very few oil glands around the eye area, making this part of the face more susceptible to signs of aging. I can recommend Microsilk-C by Raya Lab, Inc. It has a uniquely delicate under eye micro-emulsion with multi-vitamins and peptides.

Fourth Type: "Combination"

The skin may be classified as a combination of the above if some areas are oily and others are dry. These conditions may be noticeable from the chin to the bridge of the nose and across the forehead in a T-shaped form, also known as the T-zone. It is not rare to hear about men who have different conditions in different parts of their bodies, in such cases, men's special skin care products are needed to target each area.

Fifth Type: "Sensitive"

If the skin is easily irritated when exposed to wind, cold, and sunlight, then it is the sensitive type. A man's skin type is also categorized as sensitive if it becomes irritated when using cosmetics or products after shaving. In this case, a very mild cleanser should be chosen for sensitive skin, and it should be used only at night. Extra cleansing can over-dry sensitive skin. The moisturizer for this type of skin has to contain calming ingredients like aloe vera, chamomile, calendula, and more.

Sun exposure is the primary reason for premature aging and damage to the skin. Daily sunblock has to be added to a man's skin care routine, especially if their job or lifestyle requires a lot of outdoor activities. A moisturizer with sunscreen should be considered if your male client is using any topical prescriptions for acne. For most outdoor occasions, an oil-free SPF 15 moisturizer will provide ample protection. Exposure to cold, dry air can leave the skin chapped and wind burned. In this case, a heavy moisturizer, rich in oils, will be superior over the water-based crème.

European Facial Protocol for Male Clients

The male facial technique is somewhat different than the facial for women. The differences mostly include skin products that we are going to use for the treatment and part of face to be treated. As I have previously mentioned, the male skin is somewhat different than women. The layers of skin are thicker, pores are larger, and there are more oil glands, producing more lubrication for a longer period of time. The detail extraction is one of the most important steps of the male facial since the majority of them have clogged pores.

As far as skin care products, greasy and oily products are not recommended, since I have never had any man likes the "greasy stuff" on their face. If a man has a hairy chest, it is better to skip on massaging the "décolleté" area, but it is normal to massage neck and shoulders.

> Step #1: Apply a hot towel and then cleanse.

   Firstly, apply a hot towel to soften skin and facial hair. Even if your client shaved very well, you will still feel a little stubbly on the check area. Follow with the cleanser application, using the facial cleanser application technique.

> Step #2: Exfoliattion

   Exfoliation has to be done with a skin scrub or enzymatic exfoliating mask. I can recommend Bamboo Scrub (Raya Lab, Inc.). This herbal-based exfoliating cream combines finely ground bamboo with jojoba beads and micro-fine French talc. It effectively removes dead cells off the epidermis and lifts away dull, dry skin to improve texture and appearance of the complexion. Remember, that exfoliation with a scrubbing or brushing technique is strongly prohibited for cystic forms of acne. But it is absolutely safe to use for mild and moderate acne skin conditions.

> Step #3: Steaming

   Gently remove the exfoliating mask and turn on the hot steamer, while preparing the extraction mask. My favorite extraction mask for men's skin treatment includes flaxseed meal mixed with hydrogen peroxide. Prepare it by mixing equal parts of both products before and apply to the entire face.

Leave it on while steaming the client's face. Steaming should last 5-10 min. After steaming, remove the mask with a cotton pad saturated in H2O2 3% solution and proceed with the extraction.

- Step #4: Extraction

For proper extraction, you need comedone extractor, needles, disposable cotton or gauze tissue, and hydrogen peroxide solution. I use an extractor only on hard to reach places, like nose folds, chin, inside ears, and between eyebrows. But for the rest of the face, I prefer manual extraction with my index fingers wrapped in sterile gauze. After steaming, skin pores remain opened enough that hard squeezing is not necessary. Hard squeezing traumatizes the skin and can leave marks or even scars. Instead of squeezing, rather push skin with one finger toward another. Try to remove as many blackheads and whiteheads as possible during the extraction, keeping in mind that it should not last more than 10 min. From time to time, saturate a cotton ball or pad with hydrogen peroxide and apply to the entire face. Immediately apply disinfectant solution (like Calendula lotion) on the skin if blood appears when a pustule or whitehead is removed. After the extraction, saturate the clean cotton ball with Calendula lotion and apply to the entire face.

- Step #5: Massage.

Perform a dry massage with medicated powder or talc. In my book, I am introducing several types of facial massage techniques, including lymph-drainage, anti-aging facial massage, plastic massage, and healing massage. For men's facials, you should use any massage technique that is appropriate for your client's skin type. Since most men's skin produces more oil than women's skin, I recommend using the healing massage for the majority of male facials. Men with extremely dry skin can benefit from the lymph-drainage massage, anti- aging massage, or plastic massage. Remember; do not use any greasy massage lotions; use aloe vera gel or a little massage oil instead.

This type of massage is better to do right after extraction. Put a small amount of talc or medicated powder on your hands and begin a gliding motion according to skin lines. Please, refer to the pictures above for the proper hands position.

Steps of Medicinal Facial Massage

- ➤ Step #1: Effleurage.

  A gliding stroke should be performed with tips of all fingers according to skin lines. Start with the forehead and finish at the jaw area. Repeat twice for whole face.

- ➤ Step #2: Petrissage.

  A kneading motion should be performed with index fingers and thumbs. Slightly pinch skin between index and thumb fingers, following by skin lines.

- ➤ Step #3: Kneading the nose muscles.

  The kneading is performed with thumbs of both hands, keeping remaining fingers under the chin. Duration is about 15 seconds.

- ➤ Step #4: Kneading the forehead muscles.

  Start with eyebrows, while heading up towards the hairline, slightly pinching skin between index fingers and thumbs. Repeat three times, beginning from eyebrows towards hairline; then from middle part of eyebrows to the hairline; and from the end of the eyebrows to the hairline.

- ➤ Step #5: Vibration.

  A kneading motion performed with index fingers and thumbs by slightly vibrating the skin should be performed, while pinching the skin between index fingers and thumbs. Follow skin lines and repeat 2 times by massaging whole face.

- ➤ Step #6: Percussion.

  Perform a light percussive motion with the tips of four fingers, according skin to lines, for 20 seconds.

- ➤ Step #7: Light effleurage.

  Perform a light effleurage of the whole face for about 1min. The total duration of this healing massage should be approximately 10 minutes.

In cases of mild to moderate acne, I usually follow up with a high frequency treatment. This is a very popular treatment, which may be applied directly or indirectly onto the skin to stimulate, sanitize, and heal the blemishes. The high frequency electrical current enhances blood circulation, infuses skin with oxygen rich ozone molecules, and therefore kills bacteria that cases acne. Duration of the session is 3-5 minutes. Also you can apply electrodes directly on knotty blemishes to eliminate inflammation under the skin and hold it for 1 minute for better results. Proceed with the next step.

> Step #8: Apply a facial mask.

Apply a facial mask according to the skin needs of your client, and leave it on for 15-20 min. Wash it with damp sponges or washcloths.

> Step #9: Apply a moisturizer.

Finish with a water-based or antibacterial moisturizer. In cases of dry skin, choose a light anti-aging moisturizer with sunscreen in it. The ultimate goal of any professional moisturizer is to regulate and stabilize the skin's own acid mantilla and create a very thin layer of emulsified oil-and- water protective substance. This mantle, or hydro-lipid film, varies according to skin condition and type. When a person has an acne condition, his skin has a strong acidic pH and acne products need to be alkaline to restore proper pH balance.

For acne treatment, I recommend water-based moisturizers that carry antibacterial properties as well. Vitamin B cream designed by Raya Lab, Inc. is a highly effective moisturizer for oily and blemished skin. A complex of natural botanical extracts, vitamins, and amino acids help to moisturize and balance the skin, while natural Vitamin B complex (Yeast Extract) helps to regulate oil gland secretion to reduce clogged pores and inflammations.

Shaving Tips for Your Male Client

"Shaving your face every day has an enormous impact on your skin and is, unfortunately, at the root of most specifically male skin problems. Shaving does have its advantages: by acting as a sort of mini-massage, it boosts blood circulation and increases the skin's oxygen supply. But improper shaving techniques will, over a period of time, not only nullify these benefits, but also do serious damage to even the healthiest skin. They will certainly make you look less than your best when you walk out of your door in the morning."
~Mario Badescu

In other words, shaving works as a constant anti-aging treatment by exfoliating dead cells that facilitate growth of new cells and increase blood flow that carry nutrients to the surface of the skin. But even though men have this extra, anti-aging defense in their favor, it is no reason to disregard proper care of the skin before and after shaving.

Shaving is one of the most important parts of male daily morning routine. However, not many men aware that the best time to shave are after cleansing and exfoliation the face. It will soften the skin and the facial hair, and it allows the razor to glide smoothly and safely.

It is very important to avoid cleansing and shaving with hot water. Hot water signals the oil glands to pump out more oil than necessary, which is something a man with oily skin doesn't need. While this may not be bad for dry skin, hot water causes over stimulation of blood circulation, resulting in damage of fragile blood vessels close to the skin's surface, leaving behind blotchy, couperose skin.

Instead, warm water should be used for washing the face right after cleansing and exfoliating the skin. Water hydrates the skin to ensure the blade will glide smoothly over the surface being shaved. Warm water dilates the blood vessels on the face, which, in turn, opens and relaxes pores and makes the hair follicles more pliable. Therefore, the soft hair will bend as the razor padded and allows the hair to be cut at a better angle achieving a closer shave.

The razor should be clean and the blades should be changed often if one prefers a manual blade. Nothing will irritate the skin worse than a dull blade. As for single bladed razors, they are less irritating than double bladed ones. The double bladed razors give a closer shave, but that often means really close to the skin too. For those who use an electric shaver, be sure to use pre-shave oil. The old Italian barbers would use first-pressed olive oil; today, there are many oils available from skin care manufacturers. Pre-shave oils are an essential part of achieving the perfect shave. They work to protect the skin and soften the beard.

Many men use shaving cream or shaving gel. Shaving gel probably will dry out the skin just like a bar of commercial soap. Instead, hydrating shaving cream, preferably with a high fat and glycerin content, is highly recommended. This type of shaving cream will make a good lather and protect the skin from over drying.

Needless to say, shaving has to be done in the direction that the hair grows, or more importantly, never against. Shaving across is perfectly acceptable keeping in mind that shaving too closely is the main cause of razor bumps and razor burn.

It is extremely important to remove all traces of the pre-shave and shaving cream, which if left on the skin will result in dehydration, which is one of the major causes of dull, flaky skin and premature wrinkling. A cold water splash will rinse off residue of the shaving product and will close the pores. Alcohol-free toner can be applied immediately after rinsing the face to disinfect the hair follicles.

Why is it better to avoid after-shave lotions with alcohol content? These products are dehydrating and irritating to the skin, not to mention the possibility of an allergic reaction to the color and fragrance in the product.

And lastly, moisturizing and nourishing after shaving is one the most important steps to protecting the skin from aging. Easily absorbed formula will lock in moisture, leaving skin smooth and nourished.

Using skin care products and going for salon facial treatments is no longer exclusive to women. Today, more men are aware of the significance of daily skin care routines and face protection. Dozens of leading cosmetics companies offer the best men's skin care products, men's grooming regimens, and professional acne treatments.

Our task as a skin care professionals is to educate our male clients about how take care of their skin on a daily basis. In addition, promoting regular, professional skin treatment as a necessary part of a healthy complexion is important for the modern man.

Chapter 10: Understanding Cosmetic Ingredients

Human skin contains all types of organic and non-organic substances: proteins, lipids, carbohydrates, amino acids, microelements, and macro-elements, vitamins, and water that involve multiple biochemical reactions in the cells. This process includes constant metabolism of important skin proteins, like keratins, collagen, elastin, melanin, as well as skin oil (sebum). Understanding metabolic processes in different skin layers is very important when we decide what cosmetic ingredients are most beneficial for various skin problems. For instance, Vitamin C is involved in collagen synthesis; the hyaluronic acid plays a tremendous role in skin moisturizing processes; vitamins and minerals promote skin-rejuvenating processes; water is the leading ingredient to deliver all substances deeper into skin, etc.

Many cosmetic companies do their research by looking for new ingredients that help correct sun-damaged skin, aging, and other skin conditions. And in our day, we realized that the best material for skin care is our surrounding nature that brings us simple solutions for repairing and rejuvenating our largest organ of the body. Plant extracts, natural oil, essential oils, vitamins, minerals and mineral compounds, antioxidants, organic substances, like collagen, amino acids, and peptides are mostly found in the best quality skin care lines.

Over the last decade, more skin care products have popped up using terms such as "natural" & "organic" somewhere on the product packaging. Many people are not aware that these words have little to no meaning when it comes to what they actually are putting on their skin. Just because a cosmetic product uses the words "natural" and "organic" doesn't make it safe. There is no current legal definition for the term "natural" when talking about skin care products & cosmetics. The only way to know if the product is safe is by reading the list of ingredients on the back and understanding what it particularly does to the skin.

Besides, many chemical compounds have great medicinal properties that can be very beneficial for serious skin disorders. These are substances like sulfur, camphor, zinc oxide, ichthyolum, boric acid, and more.

This chapter is dedicated to cosmetic chemistry. And the main purpose of the following material is to provide information on the ingredients that might be harmful or at least undesirable for the skin. On the other hand, this chapter contains vast material on ingredients that are most effective and beneficial for esthetic treatments. As you begin to discover and learn more about cosmetic chemistry, it becomes more apparent that you do not need to use super expensive professional skin care product lines with "millions" of serums, masks, toners, and lotions involved in a multi-step-company-designed facial treatments. The cosmetic industry makes a lot of money selling extra products for skin needs, and it becomes overwhelming for skin care specialists and for the clients as well. Believe me; the amount of money you spend on professional products has nothing to do with how effective your facial treatments are. Smart business people are looking for ways to conduct their business effectively, while keeping their overhead low.

In this chapter, I am presenting several cosmetic formulations that produce excellent results, and it is all based on formulas that I have collected for years and have tested on myself and on my clients. Most of it is very simple to prepare in the salon or at home by using natural or pharmaceutical grade ingredients. In my formulas, I use varieties of product that can be easy found in the health food stores or your local Pharmacy.

Begin to learn cosmetic chemistry by reading the product labels and recognizing what the active ingredients in the formulations that are on the market are. The listings begin with the ingredient present in the largest concentration (typically water, oil, and other vehicles) and moves downward, often ending with trace elements. You shouldn't expect an active ingredient to be in the first or second spot, but if it is near the end of a long list, it is most likely present in a very small amount. For example, Vitamin C (L-ascorbic acid) has to be at least at 10%, and alpha-lipoic acid at least at 1%. The position of the ingredient on the list can give you at least a rough idea if its concentration is sufficient. Your final step in investigating the ingredient list is to look at all (or at least the most concentrated) ingredients and make sure they are not harmful for the skin.

Undesirable Ingredients

Firstly, let me introduce several of most undesirable ingredients has found in majority of commercial skin care lines.

1. Mineral Oil

Mineral oil (paraffinum liquidum) is created from paraffin that is obtained from petroleum or crude oil. It is commonly used in cleansing creams, moisturizers, eye creams, body lotions, foundations, and other make-up applications. Despite the claim that mineral oil is among the most effective moisturizing ingredients, it is not a preferable ingredient for skin care. The mineral oil does not rinse off the skin rapidly, so build-up as a consequences can be significant. Besides, mineral oil recreates protective barriers that none of the beneficial ingredients can penetrate into skin, including water. So it basically, suffocates the skin and dehydrates it. It tends to be heavy and greasy and causes the skin to become dry or develop clogged pores. Moreover, mineral oil is allergenic and photo toxic.

Common symptoms of using mineral oil are blackheads, whiteheads, and little bumps just under the skin. However, Vaseline is a petroleum jelly, and it can be used to protect the skin from harsh, windy weather for people who have to spend a sufficient amount of time working outdoors. But for this purpose, you can use a much healthier substance like coconut oil or lanolin. It protects the skin without clogging or over drying. I will talk about this ingredient further down in this chapter. In conclusion, avoid mineral oil in your practice and your skin care line, and advise your clients not to use skin care products containing any petroleum derivative products.

2. Talc

Talc is a finely powdered native magnesium silicate, and it gives a slippery sensation to cream and powders. It is one of the main ingredients of baby powders, facial powders, eye shadows, liquid powders, protective creams, facial masks, foot powders, and face creams. Similar to asbestos, a known lung irritant and cancer-causing agent, repeated inhalation of talc could lead to talcosis. Several studies indicated that talc could lead to skin cancer if used topically. But latest research shows that there is no direct evidence was presented. Anyhow, I have found that cornstarch; powdered silk, and rice starch are better alternatives to talc.

3. Titanium Dioxide

Titanium Dioxide is an inorganic salt that is found as an inert earth mineral. It is the most common ingredient in sun blocks, tinted powders, liquid foundations, and eye shadows. It is considered to have no risk of skin irritation; however, the sunscreens containing titanium oxide are very comedogenic. It clogs the pores by reacting with skin sebum and creates blackheads, especially in T-zone area.

Avoid sunscreens containing titanium oxide. Your better choice will be sunscreens containing zinc oxide, dimethicone, salicylic acid, para-aminobenzoic acid (PABA), and natural sunscreens that include willow bark and shea butter.

4. Isopropyl Alcohol

Isopropyl alcohol is produced by combining water and propylene. Isopropyl alcohol is petrochemical substance, and it should be avoided. Like all low molecular weight alcohols, it has antibacterial properties, but it extremely dries and irritates skin, especially in higher concentrations. Latest research shows that it also can generate free-radical damage.

For the cosmetic formulations, it is much safer to use grain alcohol or ethanol. I prefer to use regular clean vodka, since it represents 40% solution of food grain alcohol. It is excellent choice for homemade herbal tinctures.

5. Benzyl Alcohol (Benzene methanol, Phenylcarbinol, Phenyl methanol)

This is a natural alcohol found in jasmine and other plants. It has been used in ophthalmic and cosmetic products. Benzyl Alcohol is an antibacterial preservative, typically used in concentrations 1 to 3%. However, it may cause skin irritation and over-drying, like isopropyl alcohol.

6. Sodium Lauryl Sulfate

This is a white powder, usually derived from coconut. It is widely used as a detergent-cleansing agent, and strangely enough, it can be found in some lotions and creams as emulsifier. This is a harsh ingredient and can strip the skin of its natural protective barrier. It even can damage the skin by cracking layers of the skin and can cause an allergic reaction for many individuals. Watch out for this ingredient on the cosmetic label and avoid using anything with it.

7. Propylene Glycol

This is a petroleum derivative, and it is widely used to retain moisture, due to its ability to attract water. It is excellent for hydrating dry skin, but it can act as a contact dermatitis sensitizer in susceptible individuals

It has been an ongoing controversy, regarding how safe this ingredient is to the skin. Latest studies have not shown that propylene glycol has any potential carcinogenic properties. But since it was not proven otherwise, this ingredient belongs as an undesirable ingredient in cosmetic product.

8. Isopropyl Myristate

This partly natural, partly synthetic chemical is used as an emollient and lubricant. This ingredient is used in almost every cosmetic line in high-end department stores. It is very allergenic and can cause some skin irritation. Besides, some studies show that it can cause clogged pores, due to its waxy consistency.

9. Isopropyl Palmitate

This is an emollient and usually derives from palm and/or coconut oil. It is undesirable ingredient in skin care product since can be very comedogenic.

10. Stearic Acid

This is a yellow substance derived from animal fat. Widely used in cosmetic as an emollient and helps keep other ingredients intact in formulation, it can produce some allergic reaction in some individuals, but generally, it is a safe product to use in cosmetics.

11. Urea

This is a water-soluble compound, related to ammonia. In cosmetic products, it is mostly used as a preservative. In small amounts, it is works as a good water-binding agent, but in larger concentrations, it may cause skin inflammation. Besides, many people have allergic reactions to the urea, especially if it used around the eyes.

12. Sodium Benzoate or Benzoic Acid

This is chemically manufactured from natural compound Benzoin. Benzoin itself is a natural ingredient that has antiseptic and antioxidant properties. Sodium Benzoate is used largely as a preservative in food and skin care. It was reported that a few cases of dermatitis occurred, while using products that contained Sodium Benzoate, especially when used around the eyes.

13. EDTA

This is a preservative (stabilizer) that is used to slow down degradation (e.g. oxidation) of ingredients by chelating (grabbing and shielding) catalytic trace metals. It is one of the most common ingredients in commercial cosmetics. It has been reported to cause contact dermatitis in some individuals.

14. Parabens (Para-Hydroxybenzoic Acid Esters)

These are food grade preservatives that are the most widely used in cosmetics. Currently, various forms of parabens are present in the food and cosmetic forms (e.g. methyl paraben, ethyl paraben, etc.). It may be potentially comedogenic and allergenic in susceptible persons. There is a fact that methyl paraben may degrade and release methanol, a potentially toxic chemical. To what degree this actually occurs in skin is unclear. Evidently, some cosmetics have start to label and develop their products as "Paraben free" to avoid any potential health issues.

15. PABA (Para- Amino Benzoic Acid)

This is a UVB blocker used in sunscreens, rarely used since 1990's. PABA can cause contact dermatitis; therefore, many cosmetic companies are avoiding using this ingredient in their cosmetic formulations.

Desirable Ingredients

The next part of this chapter is dedicated to the ingredients that may provide great benefits to the certain skin conditions, like acne, hyper pigmentation, sun damage, rosacea, and more, which are some of the most common that estheticians deal with on regular basis.

Anti-bacterial Ingredients

1. Salicylic Acid

What is Salicylic Acid? It is a beta hydroxy acid derived from the bark of the willow tree. It has a larger molecule than its cousin - Alpha Hydroxy acids. The larger size keeps them on the surface of the skin, allowing it to more effectively exfoliate upper layer of epidermis. This makes it great for acne prone skin. Therefore, salicylic acid is a perfect remedy for those who naturally have oily skin or severe acne (acne vulgaris) with clogged pores and blackheads. Salicylic acid is an excellent deep pore cleanser and an effective exfoliant, but it is also is and anti-irritant. All this properties make this product widely used for all types of skin, including sensitive type.

2. Resorcin (Resorcinol)

This is a chemical compound of the phenol group (one of the dihydricphenols). Used externally as an antiseptic and disinfectant in concentrations of 1% to 3%. And used in concentrations of 5 to 10% in ointments to treat of chronic skin diseases, such as psoriasis and eczema. A popular ingredient in some acne medications, resorcinol controls small acne lesions, and it is frequently combined with sulfur in over-the-counter products.

It is present in over-the-counter topical acne treatments at 2% concentration and in prescription treatments at higher concentrations.

3. Hydrogen Peroxide

This should really be called hydrogen dioxide (H_2O_2). Hydrogen peroxide contains one more atom of oxygen that water (H_2O) does. That makes it to be one of the most powerful oxidizers and provide powerful antibacterial properties. The most used solution is 3%, but it is also available in 35% food grade solution for internal purposes. The substance can be used in esthetic treatment as topical disinfectant and bleaching agent in higher concentrations (5-10%)

4. Grain Alcohol

This is a form of pure alcohol that has been produced by fermenting and distilling grain. It is also known as ethyl alcohol or ethanol. Besides, it being used in the production of alcoholic beverages it also used as a solvent in varieties cosmetic applications as an excellent solvent. The 80 proof alcohol, also known as vodka, is widely used for pharmaceutical purposes to obtain herbal tinctures and plant extracts. Everclear (151 proof grain alcohol) is used for many formulations in compounding pharmacy.

5. Tea Tree Oil

This is an essential oil that comes from an Australian tree called "Tea Tree" (Melaleuca Alternifolia). It has been proven to be powerful natural antibacterial and anti fungal substance. Some cosmetic companies use tea tree oil to treat skin problems like acne, athlete's foot, dandruff, and nail fungus. However, the concentration of tea tree oil in some of the formulations is not sufficient to provide antibacterial properties (e.g.1%). Concentrations of 5% to 10% are recommended.

6. Boric Acid

This is a mineral acid that usually comes in white crystalline powder form. It is widely used in ophthalmology for eye drops. In cosmetics, it can be used as astringent, antiseptic, and wound-healing substance.

Anti-inflammatory Ingredients

1. Sulfur

This is natural mineral that has a deep yellow color that has been found in the Earth's crust. In Europe, sulfur has been used as a prescription for skin problems like acne vulgaris and seborrhea. It helps to kill some species of bacteria of the skin, improving acne, seborrhea, and psoriasis. Sulfur can be taken orally as anti-acne medicine and can be added to skin care formulations.

Bio-Drying Lotion (Raya Lab, Inc.) is an effective blemish drying lotion that contains sulfur. It eliminates blemishes, reduces tissue redness, and helps to prevent acne formation. Another product manufactured by Raya Lab, Inc. is a deep pore cleansing Bio-Sulfur Facial Masque, and it contains sulfur to relieve acne and seborrhea.

2. Allantoin

This is a natural ingredient that comes in a white, crystalline, odorless powder form. Extracted from the comfrey root, it is widely used in skin therapy treatments as a healing agent, moisturizer, and effective anti-irritant. Allantoin is reported to promote skin cell regeneration and is used to treat skin ulcers, wounds, burns and sunburns, furuncles, acne, skin's abrasions, impetigo, eczema, and psoriasis.

Allantoin can also be made from uric acid, but the comfrey root type is superior. Wildly used in cosmetic industry Allantoin is one the most desirable ingredients in varieties of mask, facial cream, sun blocks, and lotions. It is considered to be nontoxic, nonirritating, and non-allergenic. The vitamin company "Now Foods" manufactures the Allantoin powder in 4 oz container that makes it easily acceptable for the public.

3. Camphor

This is a white, transparent, waxy crystalline powder with a strong aromatic odor. Historically, camphor has been in used for medicine and has been included in many pharmaceutical forms. Camphor can be naturally obtained from the wood and leaves of the camphor tree or can be synthesized from camphoric acid. Because of its antimicrobial and antiseptic properties, camphor is used in pharmaceutical compounds, personal care products, and cosmetics.

4. Ichthyolum (Ichtiol, Ichtammol)

This is brown-black liquid with a very strong smell. Ichthyolum belongs to the Petroleum derivatives and contains 10.5% organically bound sulfur. Its action on skin is prompt and useful. It's used only externally as an ointment with lanoline 20% to 50%. Over-the-counter 20% Icthyolum ointment is proven to give relief for chronic eczema and psoriasis, also for nodule-cystic acne and rosacea.

5. Zinc Oxide

This is a natural mineral that usually appears as a white powder that is non-soluble in water. Zinc oxide is a mild antiseptic and anti-irritant. When added to sunscreens, it prevents UV light from reaching the skin. Therefore, zinc oxide is very popular ingredient to protect skin from UV rays, and it is included in varieties of sun blocks. It is a safe mineral substance that, for decades, has been used to treat acne and dermatitis. If it is included in the powder, it can clear rash or irritation in a few days.

It is also the key active ingredient in diaper rash creams. It is a safe and effective ingredient, and it is usually well tolerated.

Zinc oxide ointment (20%) has been used to treat or prevent minor skin irritations (like burns, cuts, poison ivy, diaper rash, etc). Zinc oxide has soothing, healing, and drying properties.

6. Benzoyl Peroxide

This works to clear up acne by penetrating into the hair follicles to reach the bacteria that cause acne with low risk of irritation. It was one of the first agents found to be effective in treating mild acne and has been used in acne treatment for decades. Some individuals may develop high skin sensitivity to Benzoyl peroxide, especially if it is used for prolonged time. It is available in both prescription and over-the-counter forms ranging from 2.5 to 10%.

Bio-active Substances Used in Cosmetics

Bio- active ingredients are widely used in varieties of cosmetic forms, including facial creams, body lotions, and make-up and hair products. To this group of cosmetics belong water and oil- soluble vitamins, amino- acids, peptides, essential fatty acids, bioflavonoids, and antioxidants.

Many reputable cosmetic companies have been including in their products these important skin nourishment substances. For example, there is no need to tell how important vitamins for healthy skin and body. They play an important role in a metabolic processes occurring in all organs on a cellular level. Since skin absorbs all substances applying on it, oil and water-soluble vitamins can significantly benefit for skin. Water- soluble vitamins in skin care products work best in water-soluble creams and lotions. On the contrary, oil-based vitamins like D and E work great for oil-based moisturizers.

<u>Oil-Soluble Vitamins</u>

1. Vitamin A

This is a fat-soluble vitamin that is included in a vast number of cosmetic products, starting with anti-aging lines and ending acne treatment product. Retinoic acid, or Vitamin A, is well known as an effective exfoliant and has been used for years to treat aging skin. It considered a good antioxidant in some of its forms, particularly as Retinal and Retinyl palmitate. Topical benefits of Vitamin A also include its skin softening and anti-keratinizing properties and its role in maintaining soft and moisture skin help to treat some psoriatic skin disorder. As a powerful antioxidant, Vitamin A prevents Vitamin C from being oxidized too quickly. The combination of these two vitamins in creams or lotions is more desirable for skin benefits.

2. Retinyl Palmitate

This is a form of Vitamin A, and it is also known as Vitamin A Palmitate). Ester of Retinol, combined with palmitic acid, is considered a more stable alternative to Retinol for normalizing the skin's texture and helping smooth out fine lines. Studies show that it is less irritating than Retinol.

3. Retinyl Palmitate Polypeptide

This is a water-soluble formulation of Vitamin A.

4. Vitamin E (tocopherol)

This is a lipid-soluble vitamin that is considered one to the most powerful antioxidants. It is known for having a strong moisturizing agent, and it has been used for many cosmetic formulations. I recommend keeping the Vitamin E oil hand and to use it to fortify facial masks or facial lotions. In addition, Vitamin E can be used as a natural preservative, and it has been found in some natural skin care products.

The stronger the concentration of it, the better it is. I use up to 32,000IU Vitamin E oil that can be found at any health food or vitamin store. Please, use the topical version. Do not buy capsules unless you want to use it as an internal supplement.

5. Vitamin D

This is a fat-soluble vitamin. Prescription derivatives of Vitamin D are used to treat psoriasis (Dovonex). It also provides relief for certain skin problems including dermatitis, dandruff, eczema, Rosacea, and severe acne.

Water-Soluble Vitamins

1. Vitamin C (Ascorbic acid)

This is one of the most important vitamins in the manufacture of the new collagen fiber; therefore it is involved in anti-aging process. Besides, vitamin C is a very potent antioxidant. Cosmetic product with vitamin C to be applied topically is a way to directly protect skin from aging and environmental stress. Because of this benefit, the skin care industry went "crazy" with the Vitamin C products for the past decade. Millions of forms of the skin care lotions and serums were manufactured. Unfortunately, there are not many people aware that not all of them potent enough to manifest desirable effect for the skin. The reason is that Vitamin C (the form of L-ascorbic acid) is not a stable molecule when it is exposed to air and light. It will oxidize quickly under these circumstances. There is a lot of controversy going on around so-called "Vitamin C serums". Ineffective forms of Vitamin C used in those products, such as ascorbic acid and Ascorbyl Palmitate, breakdown and degrade.

The only product containing Vitamin C in form of Magnesium Ascorbyl Phosphate (water-soluble analog of Vitamin C) is highly active and stable under environmental exposure. It becomes more available to the skin if it combines with the natural lipids, like lecithin. Only a few skin care lines have effective formulas with the benefits of Vitamin C. One of them is Raya Lab, Inc, the company that developed a product called Vital Silk Serum and Microsilk-C eye cream.

Of course, the best source of Vitamin C is fresh fruit, especially citrus fruits. In fact, in fresh fruit the Vitamin C is at the peak of the potency, and it is waiting for you to prepare your own serum for the treatments. Besides, the bioflavonoids that are abundantly present in the fruits help promote effectiveness of Vitamin C. Preparation cannot be easier. Squeeze a little amount of fresh juice and apply it directly to the client's skin. It is much more effective than any commercial "magic" in a bottle.

The application of Vitamin C is an essential step as a post microdermabrasion treatment, since it promotes collagen production. For this purpose, you can use fresh lemon or orange juice (preferably organic) as a Vitamin C application. If you have no desire to mess with the fresh fruit, it is definitely your choice to use a serum that contains an analog of Vitamin C that I mentioned above.

2. Magnesium Ascorbyl Phosphate

This is a Vitamin C derivative, and it is more stable than Vitamin C. It has a comparable effectiveness as collagen synthesis booster.

3. Ascorbyl Palmitate

This is fat-soluble Vitamin C derivative. It is a good antioxidant, but it is less effective than Vitamin C for stimulating collagen synthesis.

4. Vitamin B-complex

This contains eight vitamins as well as several related substances. The group of B vitamins includes thiamine (B1), riboflavin (B2), niacin (B3), pyridoxine (B6), cobalamine (B12), folic acid, pantothenic acid, and biotin. The other related substances (choline, inositol, and para-aminobenzoic acid (PABA)) are also considered part of B-complex.

B vitamins are essential for proper RNA and DNA synthesis and cells reproduction. As our skin, hair, and nails are constantly growing and renewing, we need them to ensure the good health of these structures. Added to cosmetic formulation B-complex group of vitamins provides noticeable relief for acne, oily, or extreme dry and itchy skin. Biotin has specially known to improve acne, eczema, brittle nails, diaper rush, and hair loss.

5. Yeast Extract (extract from Brewer's yeast)

This contains a mixture of proteins, sugars, vitamins, and amino acids. Yeast extract represents full range of B- complex group of vitamins and can be added to relieve acne skin condition.

According to some claims, it may enhance the rate of renewal (cell turnover) of the skin, which provides tissue repair benefits.

6. Essential fatty acids (vitamin F)

These can be abundantly found in vegetable oils and animal fats. Olive oil, avocado, almonds, peanuts, sesame seeds contain all types of essential acids w. Topical use of essential fatty acids (linolenic, linoleic, arachidonic and oleic acids) can positively influent on metabolical processes in the skin and can provide antioxidant action.

7. Liposomes

These are an active ingredient delivery system; hollow spheres made from phospholipids (such as lecithin) that are up to 300 times smaller than skin cells. Liposomes are filled with active agents that they carry into the skin and then gradually release.

8. Hyaluronic Acid

This is natural substance that has found in joins liquid. It is sometimes referred to as a "cyclic acid". It is an effective humectants and moisturizing agent.

9. Sodium Hyaluronate

These are effective humectants related to hyaluronic acid (salt form), works to moisturize the skin.

Amino Acids and Peptides

Amino acids and peptides are bio products of the hydrolysis of proteins. Proteins like keratin, elastin, and collagen are the building blocks of skin structure. If a body is deficient on essential amino acids, it suffers varieties of skin and hair problems (premature skin aging, hair loss, and seborrhea).

The sulfur-containing amino acids, including cysteine, cystine, and methionine are essential for protein metabolism. That is why these amino acids can be found in many hair and skin product.

1. Methionine

This is an essential amino acid that normalizes lipid metabolism in the skin and can be used to treat seborrhea, photo dermatitis, skin regeneration, and hair loss.

2. Cysteine

This is an amino acid that can be synthesized in the body from methionine. It can provide some benefits to relive symptoms of seborrhea.

3. Cystine

This is the component of animal and vegetable protein. It can be added to cosmetic formulations to treat seborrhea and hair loss.

4. Tyrosine

This is amino acid that may increase the effect of Vitamin C on collagen synthesis by fibroblasts and also plays a role in melanin formation.

5. Lysine

This is an amino acid that important for collagen synthesis and is possibly ineffective when topically applied.

Unfortunately, amino acids cannot penetrate effectively into skin and are considered somewhat ineffective for anti-aging purposes. Latest research has found that peptides (a portion or building block of protein) are able to enter the cells of the skin and remain intact. Skin care with peptides is reported to reduce the signs of aging by increasing collagen production. That is why, peptides in skin care products, are now considered to be important anti-aging agent.

6. Collagen

This is the main component of connective tissue of human body. It supports skin, internal organs, muscles, bones, and cartilage. Based on this fact, many cosmetic companies are promoting their products that include collagen as a powerful anti aging remedy. But latest studies have proven that collagen cannot penetrate into skin barrier because of the size of molecules and therefore, cannot provide anti aging benefits for the skin. However, collagen can be used a moisturizing agent, due to its ability of bind water molecules.

7. Elastine

This is a fiber within the dermis, similar to collagen. It is responsible for skin texture and elasticity. In topical, it cannot penetrate the skin, but it does have a moisturizing effect.

Antioxidants

The use of antioxidants has received immense interest in recent years to protect human skin from adverse biological effects of solar ultraviolet (UV) radiation. Antioxidants are substances that destroy free radicals - damaging compounds in the body that alter cell membranes, tamper with DNA (genetic material), and even cause cells death. Free radicals occur naturally in the body, but environmental toxins (including ultraviolet light, radiation, smoke, certain prescription and non-prescription drugs, and air pollution) can also increase the number of these damaging particles. Free radicals are believed to contribute to the aging process as well as the development of a number of health problems, including heart disease and cancer.

Antioxidants in skin care are a critical component to any anti-aging routine. Topical antioxidants provide some protection against environmental damage of the skin and somewhat effective in slowing down the skin aging. Vitamin C, E, and A are generally used in many cosmetics, due to their properties to neutralize free radicals.

There are also many plant derivative antioxidants that can be found in modern skin care lines that effectively protect skin from aging.

1. Bioflavonoids

These are a diverse group of plant pigments with antioxidant properties. These substances are responsible for color in many fruits, vegetables, and flowers. As far as skin benefits are concerned, two classes of flavonoids appear to be especially beneficial: proanthocyanins (found in grapes and pine bark) and polyphenols (found in green tea).

2. Green tea

This is harvested from the upper leaves of the Camellia Sinensis plant, and it is native to the Asian countries. For centuries, green tea has been known for its anti-aging benefits and excellent antioxidant capacity. In fact, it has been proven that green tea has a significant effect on virtually everything from skin blemishes to cancers.

3. Pycnogenol

This is a water extract from the bark of the French maritime pine tree, grown on the coastal region of southwest France. It is one of the most potent, natural scavengers of free radicals. In addition, Pycnogenol restores a blood circulation in tiny capillaries of the skin. It is used in many cosmetically formulations, due to its ability to bind free radicals and protect collagen and elastin fiber from breaking down, due to harmful UV exposure.

4. Grape Seed

This extract contains bioflavonoid called Oligomeric Procyanidins, which provides fifty times more antioxidant protection than Vitamin C and Vitamin E together.

Grape Seed Extract is now becoming a common ingredient in anti-aging cosmetics, due to its high concentration of potent antioxidants. Procyanidins that present in grape seeds are also known to deliver anti-inflammatory, anti-arthritic, and anti-allergic benefits.

5. Lipoic Acid

This is a potent antioxidant that can rapidly reach and protect both water and lipid portions of skin. ALA (alpha lipoic acid) has the ability to regenerate other essential antioxidants, such as Vitamins C, E and CoQ10, which are naturally present in the cells, thus working to increase their levels. It promotes optimum efficiency for production of energy in living cells, provides natural exfoliation and inhibits cross-linking (breaking down) of collagen and elastin.

Therefore, all of the above benefits of Lipoic acid make it to be very welcoming ingredient in modern anti-aging skin products.

6. Coenzyme Q10

This is another powerful antioxidant. It helps neutralize harmful free radicals, which are one of the causes of aging.

7. Resveratrol

This is most abundant found in Muscatine grapes, which are used to make vines. It is an antioxidant that supports and protects collagen production. Studies show that it may also inhibit some mechanisms of aging by modulating gene activity.

Natural Exfoliating Agents (enzymes)

1. Glycolic acid

This is one of the members of the alpha hydroxy acids (AHA). Alpha hydroxy acids are derived from plant sources and from milk product (Lactic acid). Glycolic acid comes from sugarcane, and its unique properties make it ideal for a broad range of consumer and industrial applications. Glycolic acid is widely used for therapy of photo-damaged skin - particularly as a chemical peel to improve the skin's appearance from wrinkles, uneven pigmentation, and acne scars.

2. Lactic Acid

This is Alpha hydroxy acid, derived from milk products, and used in cosmetology to hydrate and smooth dry, flaky skin.

3. Alpha Hydroxy and Beta Hydroxy

These acids are abundantly found in many fruits and berries, including pineapple, papaya, citrus fruits, strawberry, and more. Many enzymatic skin care formulations contain papaya extract (papain) that deliver strong skin exfoliating effect.

4. Spongilla (seaweed)

This is a genus of freshwater sponges found in lakes and slow streams. Fresh water sponges suitable for skin resurfacing and provide a natural alternative approach to microdermabrasion, chemical peels (glycolic acid, Jessner's, phenol and trichloroacetic acid peels), CO2 laser resurfacing, and Erbium laser peels to correct visual facial defects such as hyperpigmentation, fine wrinkles, sun damage, superficial scars, comedones, enlarged pores, and acne scars. Upon massaging, substantially, pure spongilla powder into the skin, speckles penetrate into epidermis creating controlled microscopical injuries to the skin. By doing so, they activate a wound healing response, which normally takes place in a natural restorative response to tissue injury. Observed erythema after the application is due to the increased blood circulation in the treated skin. Increased blood circulation helps to dissolve bruises, stagnant spots and infiltrates, which make it to be a great product for acne treatments.

Therefore, spongilla speckles can be used as a resurfacing modality that rejuvenates the skin, removes old, debilitated, or dead cells from the skin's outer layer without harming the younger, living cells and result in softer, smoother skin. Besides, wound-healing responses stimulate new cell growth, increase elastin and collagen production, and improve skin tone and texture.

Herbs and Herbal Extracts

Somewhere close to five hundred of different kind of herbs and plants are used for medicinal and cosmetic purposes around the world. The majority of it belongs to the medicinal category of plants.

Along with it, many herbs have been used for cosmetics due to their unquestionable benefits. There are several classifications of herbs, according to their effect on the skin: anti inflammatory, anti bacterial, toning, calming, nourishing, bleaching, and energizing.

Here are a few of the examples of herbs that commonly used in cosmetic formulations:

Licorice Extract is a skin lightener and believed to be more potent than Kojic acid (common ingredient used as a bleaching agent in many cosmetic formulations).

Rose Hips extract is botanical extract of rose petals. Besides, the large content of rose oil that known for its superior aromas Rose Hips extract includes high concentrations of Vitamin C. It has incredible healing anti-aging and healing properties.

Witch Hazel is a well-known herb with antiseptic and astringent properties. It helps reduce excess oils and relieves acne condition, due to its antibacterial properties.

Chamomile flowers are added to facial masks to provide calming and soothing effects.

Peppermint has a cooling, soothing, and antiseptic action. This herb contains Vitamin A and C and can be used for healing and nourishing purposes.

Sage leaves have anti microbial, antiseptic, and mild astringent properties.

Calendula (flowers) is my favorite plant. Benefits include soothing, anti-inflammatory, healing, and antibacterial actions.

Comfrey leaves have the ability to heal the wounds, due to its content of Allantoin, carotenes, and mucco-polysaccharides.

Horsetail is very high in natural silica. As I mention in Chapter 3, silica is one of the microelements that is involved in keratin and collagen production. It helps to fight wrinkles and strengthen weak capillaries.

Hyssop extract is used to treat skin irritations, burns, bruises, and cold sores, due to it healing action.

Ginseng root is widely known as an excellent tonic and rejuvenator. It is used in creams, gels, tonics, and facial masks as an anti-aging agent.

Lavender flower is famous for its scent. Lavender essential oil can be added to any lotion for a unique fragrance. Besides, added to the moisturizer, it enhances antiseptic and anti-inflammatory actions for anti-acne products.

Stinging nettle contains proteins, amino acids, vitamins, and minerals and can be used as aid for anti-aging treatments. I recommend preparing infusion of this herb and adding it to facial masks as a collagen production accelerator.

Oak bark is mostly used as herbal infusion and can be used as an astringent, due to very strong tightening effect.

St. John's Wort is very popular in Europe, due to its soothing and healing properties. It also can be used as an astringent for oily and problem skin. St. John's Wort oil can be added to facial or body lotions to deliver anti-inflammatory and healing benefits.

Fats and Oils

Sebum is a complex oil that is produced by oil glands located in dermis. The main purpose of this natural lubricant is to slow down the evaporation of water from deeper layers of the skin. At the same time, it prevents excess moisture from penetrating into the skin. Skin becomes dry and flaky if it does not produce enough natural lubrication, which is very common for women of menopausal age. Consequently, the most beneficial anti-aging moisturizers have to contain not only water and water-holding ingredients, but also skin's protecting natural oils.

Some oils, like jojoba and squaline, are the most beneficial for skin's natural lubrication, since they are very similar to human skin oil (sebum).

Squalane is a lubricating oil for delicate and allergy prone skin. It is a unique, natural substance that makes up about 10% of our sebum and has been found in wheat germ oil, rice bran, and olive oil. It is known as a great moisturizer and skin soother.

Jojoba Oil is a chemically waxy ester derived from the desert plant Simmondsia chinensis. With a texture almost identical to our own natural sebum, jojoba oil is an excellent organic way to maintain healthy skin without clogging pores. Jojoba oil actually helps to balance skin's sebum, so it moisturizes dry skin and eases the oil production in oily skin.

Other vegetable and plant oils are excellent skin moisturizers that make them to be an important component of all anti-aging skin care products.

Almond oil is a vegetable oil extracted from the seeds of almonds. The oil is easily absorbable and serves as a great emollient. It is an excellent natural moisturizer that is suitable for all skin types.

Avocado oil, like olive oil, predominantly contains monounsaturated fats. The oil has various uses in modern cosmetic industry, with advantages in rapid skin penetration, and as a superior natural sunscreen. In skin care, the two major advantages of the avocado are its marked softening and soothing nature and its notable absorption. Compared with almond, corn, olive, and soybean oils, avocado oil had the highest skin penetration rate.

Cacao butter has antioxidant properties, due to tocopherols as well as certain polyphenols that suppress free radicals and soothes skin irritation. Cocoa (also called cacao butter) has been called the ultimate moisturizer and is used to keep skin soft and supple. It melts at body temperature, which is what makes it an excellent base for salon custom blending creams and lotions.

Castor oil is a vegetable oil obtained from the castor bean. It is abundant in unsaturated fats as ricinoleic, oleic, and linoleic acids. Castor oil is widely used in cosmetics for lipsticks, ointments, creams, lotions, and soaps. It has excellent lubricating qualities and is famous for treating dry skin. It is highly absorbable into skin and can be mixed with other ingredients for better penetration.

Carrot oil is a vegetable oil with an intense yellow color, due to a great amount of provitamin A (carotinoids). Added to cosmetic products, carrot oil accelerates the formation of new cells; therefore, it provides skin rejuvenation. In addition, it delivers relief for dry, chapped, and scaling skin.

Emu oil is made from subcutaneous fat of emu bird that is indigenous to Australia and is now raised on farms in the USA. As a topical application, it has the ability to penetrate skin barrier to deliver soothing, anti-inflammatory, rejuvenating and healing properties. Emu oil can be beneficial for skin problems like eczema; wrinkles, keloids, scars, and burns.

Glycerin actually belongs to the alcohol group of substances, but it has an oily consistency and is wildly used in the cosmetic industry. It can be produced from propylene alcohol or naturally from vegetable oils. Glycerin is used for decades as a solvent, humectants, emollient, and lubricant in a variety of cosmetic formulations. Glycerin hydrates and provides a natural barrier against loss of moisture from the skin. It allows topical agents to penetrate into dermis, but may clog pores when present in high concentrations. Glycerin can be found as an over-the-counter product at any drugstore.

Lanolin oil is fatty secretion from sheep's wool. It is natural substance well absorbed by the skin, and it is an excellent moisturizer and skin protector. Lanolin has great ability adsorb water, known as hydrous lanolin, which delivers excellent hydration for the dry, choppy skin. It is welcomed to many cosmetic formulations, like great emulsifier and thickening agent.

Lecithin is natural phospholipid compound containing mixture of stearic, palmic, and oleic acid, and it is also high in choline and inositol (B vitamin). Egg yolk and soybean are common source of lecithin, and it has been used in cosmetics for centuries. In modern cosmetics, lecithin is widely used as an emollient and water-binding agent.

Mink oil is a product that is rendered from the insulating fatty layer under the skin of minks. It is widely used in cosmetic products, especially in Europe, due to excellent moisturizing and skin protecting properties. Approximately 17% of mink oil contains palmitoleic acid, an essential fatty acid that is also produced by human body.

Olive oil is a well-known vegetable oil that can be very beneficial for skin as a powerful moisturizer.

Interesting fact is that olive oil can be used for dry and for oily skin to normalize skin oil production. Natural olive oil is full of antioxidants that every skin type can benefit from. Yes, even oily skin can benefit from olive oil! Oil can dissolve other oils. The olive oil mask is particularly effective at cleansing skin when combined with castor oil. The combination cleans pores and rinses dirt and extra oil away, leaving skin soft and fresh.

Rose Hip Seed oil contains a large amount of Vitamin A (retinoic Acid) and Vitamin C (ascorbic acid). It is one of the optimum substances to stimulate skin-rejuvenating processes, and it prevents the formation of scars and stretch marks. Burns, chronic skin inflammation, brown spots, dry skin, and scars (even over 20 years old) can greatly benefit from products with rose hip seed oil.

Sea Buckthorn is known in China, Russia, and Europe as one of nature's most incredible medicinal plants. Its small, bright orange berries have been cherished for centuries for their truly incredible healing, nutritive, and therapeutic qualities. The richly colored oil produced from Sea Buckthorn berries is so abundant in vitamins, antioxidants, and other healing compounds that many believe that Sea Buckthorn must have been created by some ancient plant-breeder. Sea Buckthorn berries have no match in the plant world for their content of carotenoids (pro-vitamin A), tocopherol (vitamin E), phylloquinone (Vitamin K), as well as other vitally important healing and health-promoting vitamins, fatty acids, and micro-elements. Those substances are contained in virtually every part of the Sea Buckthorn plant, including its seeds, leaves, and bark. However, the most potent concentrate of biologically active compounds is the rich therapeutic oil contained in the bright orange Sea Buckthorn fruit.

Shea butter is a natural derivative of the karite trees that grow in Western and Central Africa. Pure shea butter is a wonderful emollient that is perfect for daily use. Shea butter has a rich, luxurious texture that penetrates deep to condition and moisturize every type of skin, regardless of tone or texture. It commonly used in creams and lotion for dry and normal skin. It softens chapped skin patches, relives eczema, sunburn, smoothes stretch marks, and fresh scars.

Wheat germ oil is unrefined vegetable oil made from fresh, high quality wheat germ. It is naturally rich in Vitamins A, D, and E, and also contains Vitamins B1, B2, B3, B6, F, Essential Fatty Acids, protein, and minerals. Because of its anti-oxidant and regenerative properties, wheat germ oil is a wonderful ingredient to add to skin care cosmetics. The Vitamin E oil present in wheat germ oil promotes skin cell formation, and it is great for nourishing and rejuvenating dry, mature, and dehydrated skin, and reducing scars, stretch marks, sunburns, and damaged skin.

Essential oils are a group of oils primarily derived from plants and used in cosmetics as fragrant additives. However, some essential oils can be used as natural preservatives, due to its antibacterial properties (e.g. orange oil, lemon, geranium, eucalyptus, pines oil, camphor oil).

The essential oils most often include a mix of different chemical compounds, like alcohols, ketones, phenols, terpenes, acids, ethers, and aldehydes, which, in larger quantities, can be irritating for the skin. Most cosmetic companies use essential oils in a very small amount that can only contribute to the benefits on the formulation.

Waxes

Beeswax is a natural wax produced in the beehive of honeybees. Pure beeswax is one of nature's most perfect products for in-salon custom blending formulas. It works as a thickener, emulsifier, or stiffening agent in ointments, creams, lotions, lipsticks, and soaps.

Ceresin wax is the mineral wax, similar to paraffin. It is undesirable ingredient for cosmetic use, but some cheap cosmetic manufacturers are still using this product.

Jojoba wax beads provide gentle exfoliation without leaving micro lacerations on delicate skin. Jojoba wax produced by hydrogenating the liquid wax of the jojoba shrub to a hard white wax. These soft, spherical beads are primary used for face and body exfoliating products, and it is superior to ground nutshell or pumice powder.

Paraffin wax is the same as mineral oil, but it is in solid form. Both derived from petrochemicals, which are an extremely undesirable ingredient for skin care products.

Spermaceti is a waxy substance that is retrieved from the fatty substance in the head of sperm whales. Both sperm whale oil and spermaceti have been used as cosmetic ingredients for decades in Europe and Asia. This superior product was popular as powerful anti-wrinkle agent. Now-a-days, sperm whales have been placed on the list of endangered species, and USA government and other countries strictly forbid murdering of them. Jojoba wax is the greatest replacement of spermaceti. Cetyl esters are one of the synthetic replacements of spermaceti wax that has been successfully used for varieties of lotions, creams, body butters, and scrubs.

Other Ingredients

Water is the most frequently listed main ingredient in skin care products, used in its purest form, void of minerals and other chemicals, hence the various names like distilled, deionized, purified, etc.

Carbomers (934, 940, 941, 980, and 981) are stabilizers and thickeners commonly found in many skin care formulations.

Ceteareth are cetearyl and stearyl alcohols that are combined for use as a lubricant.

Cetyl Alcohol is a natural derivative from coconuts, and it is non-irritating and non-drying, like ethyl alcohol. It is used in cosmetics as an emollient, emulsifier, thickener, and caring agent for other ingredients.

Cellulose is a polymer of the cell walls of green plants, and it can be used as a thickener and emulsifier.

Fragrances are often an aromatic blend of natural essential oils or synthetic aromatic substances.

Guar gum is a plant-derived polysaccharide used as a thickening agent in skin care formulations. It may also increase moisture retention, due to its coating action.

Hydroquinone is the chemical compound that is used in cosmetics as skin pigmentation lightening agent. A maximum of 2% of hydroquinone is sold over-the-counter and higher concentrations (up to 6%) products are available by prescription only. The studies show that only creams with higher concentration of hydroquinone provide the desirable skin bleaching effect.

Kojic Acid is also a powerful skin lightener, and it is promoted as a bleaching agent for ethnic skin.

Kaolin (China Clay) is widely used in oil-absorbing powders and masques, because it is so highly absorbent. Clay is a must-have ingredient for salon custom blending formulations.

Nanospheres are an active ingredient delivery system. It is composed from micro-reservoir particles of porous polymers that have a special structures permitting high absorption and timed release of the agents into the skin.

NaPCA are well-known humectants, the same as Sodium PCA.

Octyl Methoxycinnamate is a UV radiation blocker that is used in sunscreens.

Octyl Salicylate is a UV radiation blocker that is used in sunscreens.

Octyl Palmitate is non-drying, non-greasy solvent; often used in cleansers, astringents.

Oxybenzone is a UV radiation blocker that is used in sunscreens.

Sorbic Acid is preservative and primarily that is used to protect products from yeast overgrowth.

Sodium Laurel Sulfate is used in most cleansers and soaps. It acts as a surfactant and offers good foaming qualities. Sodium Laurel Sulfate is a known skin irritant, but contrary to popular misconceptions, it does not cause cancer.

Xanthan Gum is natural a thickening agent.

I hope this chapter helped you to be more inclined to read cosmetic labels and understand what the benefits are of the ingredients listed on the bottle. It might also assist you to discover that the major difference between an expensive, high-end product and a lower-end one is the amount of marketing dollars spent on packaging and promotion. The majority of commercial cosmetics from department stores have some pretty effective ways of keeping the customers in the dark about what is really in their bottle. Of course, expensive cosmetic companies do not want to list ingredients or allow access to their cost. Some have label ingredients listed in barely contrasting color to the containers so they are virtually unreadable or some have too small print that you need a magnifying glass to read them. And all of them promote their products with exaggerated claims of beauty, of long-lasting effects to create an image of miraculous "stuff" that will fix skin problems right away.

After all, there is no need to spend vast amounts of dollars to realize what it will do for your skin. Read the label, and "you will be amazed how legitimate research rarely matches what a cosmetic company wants you to believe" (Paula Begoun, "Don't Go to the Cosmetics Counter Without Me", 7th Edition).

Chapter 11: Professional Ethics & Client Consulting

When I first opened my business as a full service beauty salon, I hired a full range of employees, including several hair stylists and nail technicians. Coming from a medical environment, it was shocking to realize that there were no subordination rules in the remote America's beauty world.

There were many bad experiences of having a business in a small town community, where there were not many who were familiar with the meaning of subordination to business owners. My reputation as a business owner was very weak among my employees. I was a "roommate" and equal to anybody else. If I tried establish some rules of discipline, I was treated as "bad" person, suppressing one's personal freedom. My employees felt normal to raise their voice at me, and they refused to do what I asked them to do.

Subordination is defined as quality or state of being subordinated to another, i.e. inferiority to authority or state of being subordinate to authority. Examples of insubordination include the following:

- Actively challenging or criticizing a superior's orders
- Showing open disrespect toward a higher business authority
- Ignoring rules and instructions established by higher business authority

This chapter covers the ethical issues involved in treating clients and running an esthetic business. It also gives a detailed information how establish respectful relationship with your co-workers and salon owner.

Professional ethics is one of the important aspects of building a solid business as a skin care professional, and the key to success is a quality service provided in highly professional environment. Many professional associations and organizations will have their own code of ethics, according to the specifics of the business. Beauty services also established their rules and regulations to ensure that clients and consumers are protected from improper treatment during their service.

Building Professional Relationships

If you start your carrier as an employee of an established beauty salon, you have to follow established regulations and work towards building your professional relationship with business owners and colleagues.
The following are some helpful tips to get you started in the right direction:

- Respect and conform to policies, statues, and rules established by the business owner or higher authority. Do not argue with higher authority about rules and regulations established in the salon.

- Develop a state of subordination toward the business owner or supervisor.

- Maintain effective interpersonal relationships with your colleagues and co-workers. Treat them as co-workers and as a business partners, rather than "roommates" or "school friends". Respect the work place and their work, avoiding unnecessarily criticism, especially in front of clients or other co-workers.

- Work cooperatively with your colleagues and encourage other professionals to continue improving services to clients.

- Strive to develop a positive attitude among other professionals toward clients to create an eager-to-help professional environment in the salon.

- Communication is the number one rule that comes to any understanding between you and your business partners. Keep it honest and open, listen to the other party, and maintain a friendly attitude.

- Your ideas and opinions are important, but consider another point of view to improve your services.

- Recognize and respect cultural and racial diversities among your co-workers. Never offend or abuse them based on differences in race or religion.

- Any discussion besides professional issues should be avoided during the working hours.

- Facilitate referrals to other services in the salon to help promote your colleagues.

- Be helpful and responsive to any of the needs of your co-workers.

- Be honest and accurate about your qualifications. Do not try impressing your clients by telling them about certifications that you do not have.

Opening your own business is a great opportunity to grow your professionalism and your own profitable organization. But some special skills are required to be a successful business owner. Building a strong team involves providing strong leadership, designating responsibility to the staff, setting goals, and working with your team to achieve those goals. Setting policies and procedures are the guidelines that will help you and staff to grow.

Your obligation as a business owner includes responsibility to your clients to provide the best quality services in a healthy and comfortable working environment. Part of the client's first impression of you and your business is how well the employees interact with each other. If there is one employee, or staff member, that is constantly criticizing everything and everyone, it can create an undesirable atmosphere. Working together as a team is the main goal for the success of your business.

Building Your Business with Professional Ethics

Here are some tips to build your organization with strong professional ethics:

- Use language that conveys respect for the dignity of others (for example, gender-neutral terms) in all written and verbal communication with clients, partners, and employees.

- As a business owner, value and respect your employees and treat them accordingly. Be aware of their individuality, cultures, and work specification differences, including those due to gender, sexual orientation, race, ethnicity, national origin, age religion, language, and socio-economic status. Avoid actions that are the result of unfair bias and may lead to discrimination.

- Be obligated to give reasonable critique of the professional performance of your employees. Maintain a calm and friendly attitude when it comes to any issue related to their professional performance. If necessary, take some actions in an appropriate manner to solve the problem.

- Exercise honesty and accuracy when preparing payroll for your employees. On the other hand, you are required to act trustworthy and honorable manner towards your personal.

- Take appropriate action against harmful and unethical behavior of the employees.

- To resolve ethical dilemmas and conflicts of interest, exercise a fair and straightforward approach to every detail of the matter, when either conflict arises between employees or between employee and client.

- No issues in the salon must be discussed in the presence of customers or clients.

- Be obligated to provide healthy and comfortable working environment.

Professional Ethics towards Clients

- The key elements in your relationship with the client are respect, patience, compassion, and honesty. Persons, who are seeking your service, have to unconditionally trust you in order to share their health issues and skins concerns. He or she must always know that you are willing to assist them and offer the best service.

- Maintain all information about your client with appropriate respect for privacy and confidentiality. During the consultation, be prepared that people may share many details of their lives and health issues. Never share or discuss your client's information with other people. Your client will never trust you if you talk about them to other people, because they will think you share their information with others.

- It is important that the client feel you are knowledgeable and a skillful skin care specialist. Try to show your professionalism by using medical terminology for skin disorders (i.e., better to say "acne", rather than "pimple", "pigmentation" rather than "brown spots", "milia" rather than "corn", etc.). *Suggest the treatment according the client's needs. Do not overestimate your possibilities to avoid unrealistic expectations, like promising "you are going to look 25 years younger" or "all your hyperpigmentation will be gone." It's better to tell your customer that you are going to do your best to improve their skin condition, but the final outcome may vary from person to person. Be obligated to keep your promises of trying your best.

- If you are not sure what kind of skin problem you are dealing with, honestly say so. It is better be honest than perform treatment that might harm the person. Refer the client to the competent medical authority if you are not sure if you really could help. This way, every request or situation is an opportunity to serve.

- In some cases, people do not know what kind of treatment they need to achieve results, or they might not be aware of exciting the skin problem. It will fully depend on your expertise as to suggest to them what to do to improve their complexion.

- Value and respect clients' rights to be self-directed in their decision-making in accordance with their own needs and financial status.

- Do not exercise behavior to clients, based on factors such as gender, sexual orientation, disability, religion, race, ethnicity, age, national origin, party politics, social standing, or class.

- Your physical appearance is very important for building a relationship with the client. Your appearance should always be clean and professional. I have a good habit of wearing a clean, white lab coat, because it not only helps with the initial impression, it protects your clothes from spilling lotions and creams while performing a facial procedure. Professional uniform or dress code is part of conducting good service.

- Keep your breath fresh and your hands clean. Make sure that you wash your hands before each appointment. And if you just had a lunch, make sure your hands do not have any food smell. Try not to eat garlic or spicy food that can give you bad breath during the appointment.

- Needless to say, your skin has to look its best. It is common cliché that clients always look first at esthetician's skin to make sure you take care of your own skin.

- Never be mad if a client arrives late for her or his appointment. Instead, show that you are happy to see her or him anyway even they are late.

- Never be late for the appointment yourself and arrange your schedule so that your clients do not have to wait for long time. If you are running a little late, call your client and let them know about it.

- Keep your appointment book accurate and updated. All records have to be clear and correct. Be willing to reschedule an appointment as many times as your client requests.

- Try to not talk during the treatment, unless you really need to comment about your actions or answer the client's questions related to the procedure. One of my biggest issues practicing in United States was the fact that all my clients want to talk while they are in session. First of all, it is not very appropriate for the facial treatment, since it is preferred that face remains motionless for the best result of the treatment. Secondly, the esthetician has to concentrate on the steps of the treatment, while a conversation on an unrelated subject can be very distracting.

- Many salons make their profit to sell professional skin care products to their clients. To sell, you have to have excellent knowledge of your skin care products and, most of all, believe that it really does what it promises. Do not push trying to sell your product for any means; rather explain the benefits of the skin care line in a suggestive manner. First, ask what product they are already using at home. Never try to sell a product before the actual treatment. Only upon completion of a facial procedure you should decide what product could be the most beneficial for your client's skin needs.

- Successful skin care specialists should be committed to continuously educating on new skin care technology. Stay on top of new information about products, new techniques, and newest skin care equipment, and be willing to share your knowledge with your customers.

Client Consulting

1. Begin the appointment with a new client by offering a free consultation. (I always offer a consultation at no cost. Either they will proceed with treatment or not.) Present yourself with your full name and all of your credentials. For example, you can say:" I am Samantha Smith, licensed esthetician in Colorado since December 2001" or "My name is Debbie Johnson. I am a certified microdermabrasion specialist since 2004".

2. Getting to know your client's health information is the key to a successful treatment. It will determine product choice, procedure plan, and treatment protocol. Ask your client to fill out a personal history form and client informed consent form (for microdermabrasion treatment, chemical peel, electrolysis, waxing, etc.). Two important aspects that you have to aware before begin facial procedure: 1) is there any known allergy to cosmetic ingredients or fragrance?

and 2) is there any place on their face that you have to be careful about (like in cases of facial nerve damage, recent surgery, accident, etc.).

3. During the consultation, listen to your client without interaction; make them feel that they have your undivided attention. It is a good idea during the consultation or appointment to not answer your phone; even better, turn the ring down or off.

4. While discussing client's acute skin problem, avoid the negative statements like "it is untreatable" or "you have to live with it for the rest of your life." He or she has to be convinced that there is a hope for their particular issue. Promise to do your best to help with the problem and offer your plan of the treatment.

5. Ask your client about his or her eating habits, lifestyle, and everyday stress level. The gathered information will help you decided on proper skin's treatment and design home care program according to the client's needs.

6. Share your knowledge regarding nutritional habits to help improve particular skin conditions. In most cases, skin disorders are related to the person's eating habits and lifestyle. Educate yourself in this important field of esthetics, and be ready to give complete professional advice to the client. In next chapter, I am going to provide valuable information on nutrition and supplementation for most common skin problems and conditions.

7. Discuss the cost of treatment prior the facial procedure. Nobody likes hidden charges, and it may stop a person from coming back to you. Openly speak about expected charges that they will be expected to pay. If necessary, offer you client alternative treatment at lower cost. Let the customer do her or his own choosing. For example, to treat hyperpigmentation, you can offer a series of ten microdermabrasion treatments for $95 each, or you can offer a one-time procedure of chemical peel for the cost of $105 or so. But your obligation is to let them know the details of each treatment and your preference on it.

8. During the initial consultation, you also need to examine client's skin. The Wood's lamp is one of the must-have esthetician's tools to determine client's skin type or some acute skin problems. It works on the principle that different skin conditions show different colors when viewed under the deep ultra-violet light of the lamp. The lamp works best when it operates in totally dark room, and the ultra-violet rays help you to analyze the surface and deeper layers of the skin. Different skin conditions are seen in a variety of shades; for example, the dehydrated skin looks bright fluorescent under the lamp, oily areas and comedones look yellow and sometimes pink, and pigmentation and age spots

are brown. Visual skin inspection will give you a proper idea on existing skin conditions, i.e. comedones, milia, hyperpigmentation, etc.

9. While making a skin test, you need to be aware of what the client is using for home care. Assess what product recommendation would be proper for certain skin conditions. Since not every person can afford expensive products, try to do an individual approach for every client. Students or younger clients probably cannot afford an expensive, multi-product regime. Keep it simple and suggest only cleanser, astringent, and moisturizer. Offer a sample of your product if a person uses another line, or they are not sure if they want to invest in your skin care line right away. Let them decide if the cost of the product is worth the quality.

10. Keep your clients' information well documented. As your business will grow, you will realize that it is impossible to remember all the details related to the each person. Reviewing your client's file before the appointment will always help to refresh your memory, and it can help you with all follow-up appointments.

Basic Skin Care Routine

Since esthetician often serve as client educators, communicative skills for transmitting information are essential. Another way, the information that you share with your client has to be properly understood. Explain the skin product ingredients and its benefits; emphasize the undesirable substances that some skin care product may contain.

Many customers also are not well informed on how to take care of their skins on a daily basis, and your goal as a skin care specialist is to give them complete and correct information. Explain to your client that great skin is the result of a well-thought-out daily routine that works in harmony with the natural needs of the skin.

Here are some helpful tips that can help to get your client's started in the right direction:

1. Never sleep with your make up on. It is big "NO" either for young or for mature skin.

2. Commercial soaps should be avoided for face cleaning. Those soaps have very alkaline pH, which is very drying. Use a facial wash or facial cleanser that is suitable for certain skin types.

3. Special moisturizers should be used for day and nighttime. Daily moisturizer has to have protective properties, containing sun block and humectants ingredients. Oil-based moisturizers are great for dry skin and water-based for oily. Night creams for dry and aging skin have to have nourishing, regenerative properties, but for oily and problem skin, it is best to use anti-inflammatory and antibacterial moisturizer.

4. Sunscreen should not be used every day, but only for direct sun expose. Almost all sunblock's contain sun protective chemicals that plaque skin's pores, and there is no need to put it on cloudy days.

5. Exfoliation is an essential and usage of facial scrubs is recommended at least twice per week. Even person that is seeing an esthetician on a regular basis still has to exfoliate their face between the appointments. Skin's epidermis produces nearly one billion dead cells every day, and we need to give skin a little help to clean it from its waste by exfoliating. Exfoliation facilitates new cell growth, and promotes skin care product absorption.

6. Slightly taping skin with the towel leaves on skin some moisture, which will protect skin from over drying.

7. Splashing face with cool water right after hot water helps to improve skin elasticity. Warm water opens skin pores and increases blood circulation, but cold water helps to close them.

8. A facial mask has to be a part of skin care routine. It supplies skin with vitamins and other nutrients. It gives skin extra help to restore elasticity and freshness.

9. Protection of skin not only from sun, but also from cold and windy weather helps to keep skin from aging. In this case, an oil-based daytime moisturizer is recommended.

10. Professional skin care products that can be sold only by estheticians are much more superior to commercial lines that are selling in department stores.

Traditionally, salons and spas were using exclusive professional brand-name skin care product lines. Only beauty professionals were able to purchase these products and distribute it to the customers. This process of distribution granted you a professional advantage and exclusiveness over products available in department stores. You goal is explain it to your customers while offering high quality cosmetics for facial treatments and client's home care needs.

Professional cosmetic companies usually propose a sufficient sampling program of the product as well. It allows your customers to experience the product before purchasing.

Additionally, many professional manufacturers (like Raya Lab, Inc.) offer private labeling that help you to protect your profit and your relationship with your clients. Private labeling of your skin care line is the best way to keep your business strong and successful.

In conclusion, your service as a skin care professional has to be focused on the skin health of your clients, to continuing the establishment of your relationship with your clients, and maintaining a professional and ethical work environment at all times. Your clients will be return to you and refer their friends to your excellent expertise and performance.

Chapter 12:
Nutritional Supplements for Common Skin Disorders

Your relationship with clients begins with their initial consultations, and your task as a skilled skin care professional is to help to improve their existing skin conditions. You have to show your professionalism by offering the right treatment and corrective skin product. But, no matter how powerful and effective the cosmetics that you suggested are, awareness of nutritional habits is the most important aspects to clearing skin problems.

The skin is like a mirror; it reflects everything, because it is impacted by everything, both internal and external factors. Proper nutritional and supplement regime may prevent or even reverse some skin disorders. For example, deficiencies of certain nutrients, such as Vitamin B-complex and essential fatty acids are known to cause various forms of dermatitis and other skin conditions. In many cases, simple supplements with the certain vitamins or nutrient substances can fix the problem. Some nutrients taken in doses higher than the minimal requirement (but still in the safe range) may produce skin benefits above and beyond what the basic balanced nutrition does.

You as a skin care professional have to be able give your client proper recommendations for nutritional programs and supplements that can helps to clear up some skin problems. If your esthetic course did not include information on how treat skin from the inside, you need to self educate yourself on this subject.

In this chapter, I am introducing several common skin disorders that can be controlled or even cured by dietary changes and natural supplements. Supplements include basic essential nutrients, like vitamins, minerals, and natural substances, like enzymes, nutritional oils, and herbs. Herbal remedies are increasingly popular, and now-a-days more people turn to herbal alternatives when allopathic medicine stops working.

Acne Vulgaris

Acne vulgaris is a message that something may be wrong with one's body chemistry, diet, or skin care routine. Either your client has teenage acne or your client is one whose acne skin condition persists into adult years. The dietary and lifestyle changes can make huge changes to their skin condition. Your obligation to help make them aware of it and give them professional advice on nutrients and supplements will be helpful to clear their skin.

The types of fats in their diet are a key factor for acne control. Saturated fats or partially hydrogenated fats cause damage to body tissues and promote inflammation. Partially hydrogenated oils are even worse; because they are replace unsaturated fats in cells. That type of fat has to be avoided. Food that contains saturated fats mostly comes from animal sources, like fatty meats and dairy (butter, whole milk, sour cream, and cream cheese). Low fat dairy products should be the best choice for acne sufferers. Chips, crackers, and cookies are all very high in saturated or partially hydrogenated fats. Your client with acne will to better to avoid this type of food and consume just vegetable oils, especially olive oil. The vegetable oils that are high in omega-6 essential fatty acids (corn oil, safflower oil, soybean oil, cotton seed oil) should be avoided.

Besides, alcohol, caffeine, cheese, chocolate, fried food, and soft drinks (all types of sodas) are not the types of food that should be chosen by acne sufferers. Also, all forms of sugar (candy, soft drinks, cookies, etc), and baking goods (pastries, cakes, white bread) have to be eliminated as well.

The person with Acne Vulgaris has to eat more raw vegetables and maintain a high-fiber diet. This helps to eliminate toxins from the body and maintain healthy intestines. In order to prevent inflammation, it is important to add sufficient amounts of protein to the diet and cut out carbohydrates.

Eating green veggies, whole grains, fruits, low fat dairy, lean meats, fish should be the basic of anti-acne nutritional regime. The more natural food will be consumed, the faster the skin will heal.

In most cases, Acne Vulgaris is caused by hormonal imbalances. Over production of the hormone testosterone in young people is the major factor causing teenage acne. Proper hormones metabolism can diminish acne symptoms and reduce breakouts. The organ most responsible for illuminating excess of hormones and clearing them from blood stream is the liver. A liver that is not performing at the best it can worsen acne, because it cannot properly break down excess hormones from the body that it should. Maintaining healthy liver function promotes healthy skin; therefore liver support remedies have to be added to an acne treatment program.

Simple ways to clean the liver is by drinking plenty of water with fresh squeezed lemon. Personally, I recommend it to all of my clients, because it is a very easy method that can clear up breakouts and promote a healthy complexion. The lemon water should be prepared daily by adding slices of lemon to drinking water.

Nutritional Supplements for Acne

These can significantly decrease inflammation and infection. The most beneficial vitamins and minerals for acne eruptions are Vitamin A from fish oil and Zinc.

- Vitamin A is necessary for skin healing. The dose of 25,000IU per day is usually recommended to be for three months. After visible improvement, the dose can be decreased to 10,000IU daily.

- Vitamin E promotes healing processes, and it is recommended that it be taken orally at doses of 400IU per day. Vitamin E is a potent antioxidant that enhances tissue repair; therefore, it can prevent acne scars formation.

- Vitamin C promotes immune system strengthening and helps fight inflammation. It is also plays an important role in collagen production and can promote healing of post-inflammatory scars. Vitamin C should be taken daily in the amount of 500-1,000mg.

- Omega-3 fatty acids (fish oil, flaxseed oil and primrose oil) have antibacterial and anti-inflammatory properties and can be added to the anti-acne diet for tissue repairing, healing, and unclogging the pores. The method of use usually indicated on the bottle. Usually one or two capsule per day is recommended.

- People with acne usually have some digestion problems. Adding probiotics to the diet will replenish healthy bacteria to reduce outbreaks.

- The group of B-vitamins is one of the most important supplements that have to be taken by person from mild to severe acne skin problem. Vitamin B2, (riboflavin), Vitamin B3 (niacin), Vitamin B5 (pantotenic acid), Vitamin B6 (pyridoxine), folic acid, and biotin are the most beneficial ones that are recommended for acne sufferers, B3 (100mg three times a day), B6 (50mg three times a day, B5 (50mg three times a day). However, it is recommended to take B-complex vitamins since as a group it will work more beneficially. The recommended dose is 100mg two or three times daily.

- Zinc is a mineral with antibacterial properties. A diet low on zinc promotes flair-ups. People with acne problems have to take a zinc supplement in the amount of 30-80mg per day.

- Chromium picolinate helps reduce infection of the skin and should be taken as directed on the label.

- Colloidal silver is known as natural antibiotic and has been successfully used for different types of bacterial and viral body problems. It can be added to someone's diet that is suffering from acne vulgaris.

Certain herbs can be added to the dietary supplementation for acne healing. Creating a skin care regime that includes herbal supplements will lead to healthier skin overall.

- Goldenseal contains a compound called berberine that kills many types of bacteria, including the ones that cause diarrhea. Berberine has also been shown to kill a wide range of other types of germs, such as those that cause candida (yeast) infections, viruses, and various parasites, such as tapeworms and Giardia. Berberine may also activate white blood cells, making them more effective at fighting infection and strengthening the immune system. For these reasons, berberine is used as an antibiotic and disinfectant, both externally and internally. In order to clear up acne skin problems, Goldenseal as a supplement is available in tablet and capsule form and has to be taken orally at recommended dose for 2-3 months.

- Important steps for acne recovery include an herbal liver and blood cleanse. As I mentioned earlier, the malfunction of the liver may cause hormonal imbalance that leads to skin breakouts and clogged pores. Burdock root, Dandelion leaves, Milk thistle, and Red clover work as a blood and liver purifiers. Burdock root and Dandelion help to eliminate toxins from the body by improving liver function. They contain natural insulin that helps to fight bacteria that cause skin inflammation.

- Adding Chaste tree berry extract can aid in preventing premenstrual breakouts.

- Neem is one of the most powerful blood purifiers and detoxifiers in Aurvedic medicine. Due to its antibacterial properties, it can effectively fight the common epidermal dysfunctions, such as acne, psoriasis and eczema. The recommended dose is 1-2 capsules twice per day after meal.

- Turmeric is especially useful for the treatment of certain skin disorders, such as acne, when administered orally. It is a wonder herb that has multiple benefits for the body. The active ingredient in Turmeric is curcumin, and it has antioxidant, anti-inflammatory, and has antibacterial properties. The antibacterial properties help to restore the skin's natural balance, while eliminating harmful bacteria that cause acne and acne rashes. This supplement is wildly available in any vitamin or herbal store and has to be taken at the recommended dose.

- Licorice root extract possesses a natural anti-inflammatory agent that can soothe the skin affected by blemishes. It is also assists in limiting of the production the irritants of the body that contribute to the formation of acne.

Modifying dietary habits and taking nutritional supplements are not only options that can help for acne skin problems. Stress reduction, regular exercise, and sunshine also can facilitate healthy skin restoration. All this recommendation has to be given to client who is seeking help for acne skin disorder. Proper diet, nutritional supplements, esthetic acne treatments, and proper skin care products are all needed to correct the problem.

Rosacea

Dietary changes are extremely important in helping to reduce the symptoms of rosacea skin condition. By simply avoiding certain foods that causes flare-ups may enhance esthetic Rosacea skin treatments and get your client on the road to recovery much faster.

Diet plan for clients with Rosacea should include adding food rich in omega-3 essential fatty acids. Certain types of fish like halibut, mackerel, salmon, and sardines have a sufficient amount of Omega-3. Supplementation with fish oil can be added for extra support.

Raw or cooked vegetables, fruits, low fat dairy, lean poultry, whole grains, and beans are going to be an excellent choice for rosacea sufferers. The troublesome products, like alcohol (especially wine, coffee, aged cheese, spicy food, fried food, sugar), have to be avoided because they may cause flushing. Lifestyle habits, including saunas, hot tubs, extreme exercise, and stress can worsen the symptoms of rosacea.

Some recent studies show that people with rosacea can significantly benefit from alkaline diets that include alkaline pH food.

Here is complete list of alkaline food that is preferred for people with rosacea:

Vegetables: Asparagus, Artichokes, Cabbage, Lettuce, Onion, Cauliflower, Radish, Peas, Red Cabbage, Leeks, Watercress, Turnip, Chives, Carrots, Green Beans, Spinach, Beets, Garlic, Celery, Green grasses (wheat, kamut, barley), Cucumber, Broccoli, Kale, Brussels Sprouts

Fats and Oils: Flax, Hemp, Avocado, Olive, Evening Primrose, Borage oils

Fruits: Lemon, Lime, Tomato, Grapefruit, Watermelon, Rhubarb

Drinks: fresh vegetable juice, pure water, lemon water (pure water and fresh lemon or lime), herbal teas, vegetable broth, non-sweetened soy and almond milk

Seeds, Nuts, and Grains: Almond, Pumpkin, Sunflower, Sesame seeds, Flax, Buckwheat, Spelt, Lentils, Any sprouted seeds

The key supplement for Rosacea is zinc. Digestive enzymes, Vitamin B-complex, and liver cleansing herbs like Burdock root, Red clover, Dandelion, and Milk Thistle can be added to the diet to improve Rosacea skin disorder as well.

According to some studies, people with Rosacea do not produce enough of hydrochloric acid naturally occurring in the stomach. Supplementation with hydrochloric acid (600mg) with each meal can reduce the symptoms of rosacea like redness and flashing. The course of treatment with these supplements has to last from 3 to 4 months until significant improvement occurs.

Dermatitis

When it comes to skin, the single most important B vitamin is Biotin, a nutrient that forms the basis of skin, nail, and hair cells. Without adequate amounts of this vitamin in the diet, person may end up with dermatitis (an itchy, scaly skin reaction) or hair loss; therefore, supplementation with Biotin can help to improve dermatitis skin condition and other skin disorders.

Seborrhea Dermatitis (Seborrhea)

The majority of people with seborrhea have digestive system disorders that lead to hormonal imbalances, weak immune systems, and chronic infections. Strict diet is strongly recommended for the clients who have this skin disease. Importantly, all animal fat has to be eliminated from their diet. Low fat proteins like poultry, fish, and lean beef have to be chosen over pork and fatty beef. Sugar, chocolate, whole dairy products, white bread, cookies, and fried food should be avoided. Dairy products have to be consumed in moderation only having preferences for yogurt, low fat milk, and low fat cheese.

Supplemental program should include essential fatty acids (evening primrose, fish oil), Vitamin B-complex in dose of 100mg per day plus extra B6 vitamin in dose of 5 mg three times per day and Biotin (300-400mcg 3 times per day). Zinc has to be also added to strengthen the immune system and to facilitate healing processes.

Colloidal silver is a natural antibiotic that has been known for it excellent properties to fight bacteria, and can be added to the supplemental program for Seborrhea sufferers. Olive leaf extract is also known as beneficial herb to treat seborrhea, because it has healing properties.

Acidophilus has to be taken every day to replenish "friendly" bacteria and support intestinal flora. Along with the dietary changes and nutritional supplementation, lifestyle changes can bring outstanding results to relieve Seborrhea. Stress has to be avoided by means of stress management techniques like yoga, meditations, moderate exercise, etc. Calming herbs like Valerian, Chamomile, and Kava can be taken to relieve anxiety and stress.

Eczema (atopic dermatitis)

This is the skin disease that can be reduced with proper treatment, though the skin will always be sensitive to flare-ups and need extra care. Allopathic medicine treats eczema with steroid creams that might temporary give the relief but do not eliminate the cause.

Correct dietary supplementation can reverse eczema symptoms of people who suffer from this skin disorder for years.

Diets high in fiber with lots of fresh vegetables are the key to clearing and preventing eczema flare-ups. The nutritional program should contain low-fat protein, low-fat fermented dairy (if one does not have lactose related allergy), gluten-free bread, whole grains, and apples. Fruits with high glycemic index have to be avoided. Eggs, sugar, chocolate, peanuts, and wheat have to be eliminated from some people's diets as well. Not to mention, that soft drinks have to be substituted with drinking a sufficient amount of drinking water.

Colon cleanser with herbal or fiber supplementation should be used as an aid for toxin removal from the body.

Some additional supplement that may contribute to Eczema symptoms relief:

- MSM is effective supplement for treating certain skin disorders and can be added to people's diet who suffers from eczema. It reduces inflammation and contains natural analgesic.

- Vitamin B-complex, taken in doses of 50-100mg per day, relieves stress that often aggravates eczema. Besides, this supplement is essential for healthy skin and proper blood circulation. For faster symptoms' relief additional doses of Vitamin B3 (100mg), Vitamin B6 (50mg), and Vitamin B12 should considered for severe symptoms for eczema.

- Biotin belongs to the Vitamin B-complex and has to be added in dose of 300mg daily.

- Vitamin E relieves itching and dryness and can be used both topically and orally. Recommended dose is 400IU per day or topical application with Vitamin E oil, containing 32,000UI of Vitamin E.

- Vitamin C with bioflavonoids inhibits inflammation and restores healthy tissue.

- Vitamin D3 also has a soothing effect on tissue and should be added to the nutritional program in doses of 400-1000IU daily.

- People with skin conditions, such as eczema, often have fatty acid deficiencies, which may lead to the onset of the condition. Therefore, adding essential fatty acids to the diet can relieve itchiness and skin irritation. By providing moisture to the skin, essential fatty acids prevent dryness and flaking.

- Lecithin also can help to improve dry skin and provides long term moisturizing benefits.

- Brewer's yeast can be added to the diet to promote healthy skin since it contains mostly all B vitamins.

Herbal supplementation should contain herbs that support liver function and have blood-purifying properties. Dandelion, Red Clover, Goldenseal, and Myrrh can be used in capsules or tea form.

- Red Clover is a member of the pea family and contains tocopherol, a powerful antioxidant that helps destroy toxins. Red clover alleviates eczema and other chronic skin conditions.

- Chamomile can be taken internally or used topically as herbal infusion to sooth the skin and reduce inflammation.

- Grape seed extract contains oligomeric proanthocyannodinc that reduces inflammation and removes toxins that cause eczema.

Psoriasis

Dietary changes should be first taken into consideration for psoriasis healing program. The diet has to be composed of 50% raw foods and include fruits, grains, and vegetables and, as a source of protein, the best choices are fish or lean poultry. Avoiding refined sugar products, fried and processed food are a must.

Bowel and liver cleansing is extremely important part of every prevention or curing program. Our internal organs can hold a lot of toxins that can cause skin problems like psoriasis and eczema. Your recommendation to the client with such a skin condition has to include herbal liver cleanse and bowel cleansing fiber. Many fiber components, such as apple pectin and Psyllium husks, are able to bind to bowel toxins and promote their excretion.

Refer, to the information above on liver cleansing herbs. In addition, Sarsaparilla and Yellow Dock herbs are also known as good liver detoxifiers. Lavender is good to use for bath or sauna. It soothes and heals irritated skin.

Psoriasis skin condition can also benefit from sunlight exposure and a low stress lifestyle, since it is known that symptoms of psoriasis can be triggered by nervous tension. Exposure to the direct sun for fifteen minutes to half an hour may reduce the scaling and redness of the skin.

Essential supplements for psoriasis relief include Vitamin A, Vitamin D3, Vitamin B-complex, Vitamin E, zinc and Copper. Copper is a microelement that balances zinc and has to be taken up to 3mg per day, while zinc doses contain 50-100mg daily.

Essential fatty acids have to be added as secondary supplements to moisturize the skin from within. Dry skin conditions, such as psoriasis, are often a sign of fatty acid imbalance. Your skin cells need to have healthy cell membranes to prevent moisture loss, capture nutrients, and keep toxins away. Fatty acids are necessary for this and to help keep skin cells strong and functioning properly. Great source of Omega-3 is flaxseed oil, evening primrose oil, and fish oil and has to be taken as directed on the label.

Also supplement like MSM can be helpful in tissue repair and reducing inflammation. The dose should contain 500 mg per day.

Some studies show that supplements with grape seed extract (300mg daily) and olive leaf extract (1000mg daily) give great results for relieving psoriasis symptoms.

Along the same lines, the selenium and Vitamin E combination may benefit people with other types of skin inflammation too, such as psoriasis, dermatitis and eczema. Daily supplemental dosage is 50 micrograms once or twice per day.

Dry Skin

The environment, the time of the year, and even age can contribute to dry skin. Internal causes of dry skin include reduced oil gland function and poor diet. Reduced oil gland function results in a reduction of lubrication available to the skin. This lack of lubrication increases water loss on the skin's surface and leads to dehydration, which leads to dry, flaking skin.

Poor diet or a diet low in healthy fats and high in processed foods and sugar, leads to deficiencies in water intake and supplements with vitamins, minerals, and essential fatty acids can support smooth, supple skin. In addition, a diet with sufficient water intake can to help promote healthy gland function and help skin retain its optimal moisture levels.

Here are some dietary suggestions to relieve symptoms related to dry skin:

- Maintain a balanced diet that includes vegetables, fruits, grains, seeds, and nuts containing certain amounts of quality protein from animal or vegetable sources. Foods such as garlic, onions, eggs, and asparagus are high in sulfur and adding them to the diet helps to keep the skin smooth and youthful.

- Increasing essential fatty acids is important for efficient skin lubrication. Cold-water fish, walnuts, and flaxseeds are all rich sources of Omega-3 fatty acids, which can help replace moisture in dry hair and skin. Also, unrefined, cold-pressed flaxseed oil should be use daily on salads, or mixed into any dishes. Flaxseed oil contains great amounts of Omega-3 (alpha linolenic acid) and Omega-6 (linoleic acid). These are converted in the body into hormone called prostaglandin, which support skin health. Fish oil contains efficient amount of omega-3 as well and can be supplemented on daily basis for amount of 1000-2000mg. When a person ingests these essential fatty acids, which human bodies need but don't make, they form healthy cell membranes that can effectively hold water inside the cell. The more water in the cell, the better hydrated the skin.

- Evening primrose oil is a supplement that is very beneficial to treat dry skin. It contains gamma-linolenic acid (GLA), and other essential fatty acid reputed to strengthen skin cells and boost their moisture content. It comes in capsules, and the recommended daily dose is two 500mg capsules, three times daily.

- Fruit and vegetables that have orange, red, or yellow color are high in beta-carotene (Vitamin A). Vitamin A is an antioxidant that promotes cellular repair and is necessary to improve dry skin conditions. Cantaloupes, carrots, and apricots are healing foods for dry skin, because they are rich in the Vitamins A and C, both important to maintain moisture in the skin. Eating food rich in pantothenic acid (Vitamin B5), such as raw milk, cheese, natural plain yogurt, kefir, leafy green vegetables, nutritional yeast, and wheat germ, support synthesis of fats and oils used by the skin.

When feeding skin through a healthy diet, it is the best to focus on its hydration. Drinking at least 2 quarts of quality water every day will keep the skin well hydrated. One also has to choose water-based fruits and vegetables. This category includes food like cantaloupe, grapes, oranges, celery, cucumbers, tomatoes, green peepers, and onions.

To improve dry skin condition, it is essential to avoid fried foods, animal fats, and heat-processed vegetable oils. The preference should be given to cold-pressed oils only. Heating oil leads to the production of free radicals that produce damage to the skin. As well as products like soft drinks, refined sugar, chocolate, alcohol, and caffeine should be eliminated from one's diet. Coffee and alcohol are the number one substances that have to be avoided since they have a diuretic effect, causing the body and skin cells to lose fluids and essential minerals.

Supplements for Dry Skin Condition

- Fish oil -Take 500 to 1,000 milligrams of fish oil daily. If you have extra-dry skin and consume fish, up the dose to 2,000 milligrams a day.

- Vitamin A deficiency can lead to skin-related symptoms, including a dry, flaky complexion. That's because Vitamin A is necessary for the maintenance and repair of skin tissue. Adding Vitamin A to one's diet is essential to restore dry skin.

- Vitamin B-complex is also helpful supplement to relieve dry skin. To elevate the unpleasant symptoms, one should add extra Vitamin B12 (100mg 3x daily) and Biotin (300mg per day).

- Vitamin E should be taken at 400-800mg IU 4x daily, as well as zinc (50mg 4x daily).

During the initial consultation, you have to educate persons who suffer from dry skin condition about how to take care their skin on a daily basis. One should not use hot water to wash his or he face, since it can lead to over drying the skin and commercial facial soaps have to be mandatorily avoided. As I have mentioned previously, soaps have very alkaline pH and can easily throw someone's skin out of balance. Consequently, this can cause many uncomfortable symptoms associated with dry, flaky skin. It is better to use lukewarm water with a mild facial cleanser with balanced pH. It is also important to introduce to your client how to properly moisturize the skin. It is more efficient to apply the moisturizer while skin is still wet, in order seal in the moisture.

Oily Skin

Most people experience oily skin when they hit puberty, and hormones begin to rampage across the bodily systems. Causes of oily skin have also been attributed to diet, stress, and environmental issues, but the main reason for oily skin is the increased production of skin oils, or sebum, usually associated with hormonal changes. People with oily skin are more prone to develop Acne Vulgaris than any other type of skin. Often, chronically oily skin has enlarged pores, comedones, and pussy pustules. The skin looks shiny, thick, and dull colored.

A smart diet and proper supplementation can really control excess oiliness. It is very important that someone completely avoids greasy and starchy foods, as these will directly contribute to an increase in oil. Instead, vegetables and fruits can be added, as many as five daily servings, for someone's diet that suffers from with oily skin. Fiber-rich foods, such as complete grains, should also be included. Dairy products are high in saturated fat that make the skin oily, causing skin outbreaks and worsening acne; therefore, dairy, like cheese and whole milk products, should be excluded from their diet. Avoiding refined sugar, cakes, pastry, alcohol, and soft drinks that high in sugar can significantly improve oily skin conditions. But junk food, like chips, high fat, high-salt food, like burgers, and other fried foods may impact the skin as they do entire body. Grilled or steamed foods are therefore recommended over fried foods.

Another important factor to be included in the diet for people with oily skin is water. Drinking 8 glasses of water a day hydrates the skin, keeping it healthy and moisturized. Water is considered the healthiest way to treat acne-prone skin with the added benefits of maintaining a healthy body. Drinking 8 glasses of water per day can also delay the signs of skin aging as well.

Supplementation regime to improve oily skin is the same as for acne skin disorder. Vitamin B-complex, essential Fatty acids, Vitamin E and A, and zinc are essential for sufferers of oily skin. Please, refer to the information above for the recommended doses of the supplements.

Home care regime has to include washing the face twice per day using a cleanser for oily skin. Harsh or drying cleansers are not recommended as this will cause a "rebound reaction" in which oil glands are forced to work overtime in an attempt to counteract the dryness, caused by these type of cleansers.

After thoroughly washing the face, an astringent or toner has to be used to close the pores and remove excess of oil. In severe skin oiliness, an astringent is recommended up to 4 times per day, especially if the person sweats a lot after performing some physical activities. Next step is a moisturizing. Preference should be given to oil free or water–based moisturizers that have antibacterial properties. The moisturizer can be used in the morning and at night.

Anti-Aging Nutritional Program

Beautiful skin is achieved from inside and out, and a healthy diet goes side-by-side with the anti-aging skin care routine. Foods with refined sugar and refined wheat can produce hyperglycemia (a sudden rush in the blood sugar levels) that promote inflammation and promote skin aging. It is estimated that approximately 50% of all skin aging is caused by sugar-induced hyperglycemia.

In addition, refined sugar and carbohydrates (such as refined wheat) converted to sugar have a specific detrimental effect upon collagen causing cross-linking and a loss of elasticity. The result is the promotion of sagging skin and premature wrinkles. Cutting out sugar and white bread and adding wholesome fresh food are an integral part of ageless skin.

Certain foods slow down skin's aging and have to be considered to adding to one's diet. Food such as raw nuts, green leafy vegetables, seeds, seaweed, barley greens, and olive oil are said to help with regeneration, which is when replicated cells are stronger than the dead ones being replaced.

Protein is the key of healthy diet and becomes even more critical, starting in the 40s, when muscle mass begins to decline by up to 1 percent a year. To combat the aging process, it is recommended to eat plenty of skinless chicken and turkey breast, lean beef and pork, eggs, beans, and seafood.

The free radical theory of aging has been the subject of scientific research in recent years. It has been proven that consuming sufficient amounts of antioxidants slows down the aging process of the human body. Between birth and approximately age 27, the body's antioxidant integrity is equal to or greater than the body's free radical activity, and there is less cell damage during these years. At age 27 and beyond, the antioxidant integrity declines below the level of free radical activity and damage progressively increases in volume, as a person ages. By age 82 it is estimated that the process of free radical damage is 60 times greater than at age 22. Accordingly, an anti-aging diet should contain a sufficient amount of antioxidants and Omega-3 fatty acids; therefore, fresh fruits, vegetables, and healthy fat have to be given dietary preferences. The potential to enjoy a healthful and active life is greater for people who eat an antioxidant rich diet, than for people who do not.

Unfortunately, as person ages his or her body does not assimilate nutrients as well as it did in younger age. The right supplements and nutrients have to compensate for the deficiencies that occur in organisms. Any anti-aging program has to include supplementation with powerful antioxidants, like Vitamin E (600mg per day), Vitamin C (up to 1000mg once per day), Lipoic acid (200mg per twice per day), and DMEA (250mg twice per day).

As I have mentioned earlier, **Vitamin C** promotes proper collagen metabolism and has to be used internally and externally on daily basis. Besides, it is an antioxidant that helps protect skin from the damaging action of free radicals; it also is a powerful aid in tissue healing and repair. Excellent sources of Vitamin C include vegetables, like leafy greens (lettuce, spinach, parsley, mustard and turnip greens, and kale). Also, cruciferous vegetables, such as broccoli, cauliflower, cabbage, and Brussels sprouts, and familiar citrus sources, such as oranges, lemons, and grapefruit, contain sufficient amounts of Vitamin C. It is beneficial to supplement with Vitamin C in capsule form or powder form, but a natural source is always more preferable.

Vitamin E helps to fight cellular aging by protecting cell membranes. Dose of 60 mg per day is recommended.

Another powerful antioxidant and aid in proper blood sugar balance is **Alpha-lipoic acid**. This powerful antioxidant is hundreds of times more potent that either Vitamin C or Vitamin E. What makes it so special is its ability to penetrate both oil and water, affecting skin cells from both the inside and the outside of the body. Alpha-lipoic acid can be taken as a supplement in capsule form and topical cream, and it is a superior aid to cellular protection.

DMAE (dimethylaminoethanol) is a powerful antioxidant. This nutrient has one of the strongest appetites for free radicals, and it prevents formation of lipofuscin. The lipofuscin is a byproduct of free radical damage in skin cells.

The formation of lipofuscin is associated with a deficiency of some important nutrients, including Vitamin E, selenium, glutathione, chromium, and dimethylaminoethanol.

Grape seed extract is also one of the powerful antioxidants that help prevent age spots formation.

Green tea contains polyphenols, which is one of the most powerful natural antioxidants. Green tea appears to exert sun damage protection by quenching free radicals and reducing inflammation, rather than by blocking UV rays. Green tea is known to benefit the skin in almost every way, leaving face and body looking healthy, young, and smooth.

Aging is generally associated with decreases in tissue **CoQ10,** a naturally occurring compound that plays a key role in producing energy in the mitochondria. For example, levels of CoQ10 in the skin are low in childhood, reach a maximum at around 20-30 years of age, and then decrease steadily with increasing age. Supplementation with CoQ10 may dramatically decrease skin's sign of aging and protect from future deterioration. The CoQ10 can be found at any vitamin store and has to be taken in doses as directed on the label. CoQ10 is found in some foods such as fish and meats.

Essential Fatty acids, like fish oil, borage oil, and evening primrose help to enhance the skin's natural moisture, increase elasticity, and provide a healthy glow. Recommended dose is 1-2 capsules per day, containing 1000mg of oil.

Hyaluronic acid is a natural substance that is present in synovial joint fluid and in the dermis, but it diminishes with age. If it were not for the tremendous water binding properties of hyaluronic acid, the water would flow from human's eyes. It is an important supplement for men and women, who are beginning to see the first signs of skin aging. The hyaluronic acid moisturizes skin from inside out, smoothing the wrinkles and fine lines. For anti-aging properties, it advised to take orally at recommended dose for two or three months. Hyaluronic acid, combined with essential fatty acids (building blocks), helps to repair the skin and diminish fine lines.

Copper is an important mineral to fight the signs of aging. Together, with Vitamin C and zinc, copper helps to manufacture elastin, the fibers that support skin structure from underneath.

Selenium (200mcg) is a trace mineral that helps to boost the immune system and fight off infection, providing a general increase in the body's defense against dangerous bacteria, viruses, and cancer cells. Anti-aging benefits of selenium are tremendous, since it works as a skin defender against free radicals.

Couperose Skin (telangiectasia)

Human skin undergoes numerous visible changes as it starts aging. Brown stops (age spots), saggy skin, baggy eyes, and wrinkles around the eyes and mouth are all results of body aging process. Two of the most prevalent damaging aggressions are UV exposure and temperature extremes. UV rays accelerate the deterioration of the skin's elasticity in general and the capillary elasticity as well. Couperose skin, also called telangiectasia or diffused redness, is a widespread skin disorder, frequently encountered by the estheticians.

Couperose skin is characterized by the visible presence of capillaries, bright red in color, winding delicately through the tissues around the nose, on the cheeks and the chin. Diffused redness, frequently precedes the appearance of couperose, is a constant flushed appearance of the cheeks and nose. Therefore, the skin that is covered with small broken capillaries (telangiectasia) is called couperose.

As women age, they begin to lose the hormone estrogen that causes thinning of the epidermis. Tiny capillaries underneath skin become more visible and create an unpleasant look. Consumption of alcohol, tobacco, and caffeine can dramatically increase this process. Besides, walls of capillaries become weaker and can break very easily, creating so-called "angiomas".

Climate conditions and harsh weather particularly wind and cold, contribute to the couperose condition as well. Especially damaging are sudden changes in temperature, like going from a warm room into the freezing cold wind outside. When the skin is very warm, the capillaries dilate, bringing blood to the surface to cool the body. The sudden shock of piercing cold causes the capillaries to constrict. This repeated dilation and constriction overtax their elasticity. Similarly, overuse of a sauna, long hot showers and very hot water on the face should be avoided on a very delicate skin.

For such a person lifestyle and habits can be the skin's worst enemy. In fair, delicate skin, predisposed to couperose, a steady diet of hot, spicy food, chronic alcohol consumption and eating meals too quickly will promote couperose. Then, there is cigarette smoking, which depletes Vitamin C in the skin, essential for the formation of collagen, and accelerates the cross-linkage of collagen and the hardening of elastin, and furthermore, it creates a trillion free radicals, which destroy the capillary structure.

Diet plays a pivotal role in caring for couperose skin. One should have a diet with skin-replenishing antioxidants, such as Vitamins A, C, E, and B-complex, including Biotin. Fish oil, flaxseed oil, and evening primrose oil, which supply essential fatty acids, help strengthen cell walls and blood vessels.

Also of interest is Vitamin P, so named because it increases permeation of gases and fluids across circulatory vessel walls. Vitamin P, otherwise known as bioflavonoid, enhances the use of Vitamin C by improving absorption and protecting it from oxidation. A great source of this substance is found in the edible pulp of fruits, green pepper, broccoli, and red wine. The Vitamin P promotes blood vessel health and improving capillary strength. It has anti-inflammatory properties and helps protect against infection and blood vessel disease.

Some herbs, like horse chestnut, are beneficial in treating capillaries or blood vessel disorders. There is interesting research on horse chestnut extract, Aesculus hippocastanum, which is rich in active substances, called esculoside, which increases elasticity and tone of the vessels, and it is a potent antioxidant to inactivate free radicals

Silica is one of the most important microelements that provide support to strengthening capillaries. Refer to the **Chapter 5: Rosacea** for detailed information on bio silicon, an important mineral that keeps bones, tendons, cartridge, and blood vessel walls healthy.

Although it might seem unsightly and frustrating, a person who suffers from enlarged skin capillaries can successfully care for couperose. Maintaining proper lifestyle, dietary program, and a carefully chosen skin care routine, anyone can really improve skin condition for a relatively short time.

The role of the esthetician begins as that of educator. Skin care specialists have to encourage the client to stay on their nutritional program and provide salon skin care treatment if necessarily. Esthetic treatments should encompass two objectives for couperose skin. First, avoid vacuum suction; vigorous brushing and other aggressive practices for a person who has couperose skin condition. Secondly, a very important objective is to use an active ingredient, which strengthens the tines of the capillary, and it is a potent antioxidant to inactivate free radicals. There are numerous products on the skin care market that help to diminish visibility of couperose. The role of the esthetician is also to recognize those skins that are susceptible to developing couperose and to advise product, especially sunscreen and treatments to maintain the healthy elasticity of the capillaries and effective circulation.

To keep the skin healthy, it is important to take good overall care of the organ, as the skin's well being is dependent on the health of the rest of body. The diet and lifestyle habits that support healthy skin include high- nutrient, high-water-content and high-fiber- content food. Supplements for healthy skin include a multivitamins, minerals, antioxidants, and the essential fatty acids. By sticking to these simple rules and working in conjunction with an experienced skin care specialist, many common skin care problems can be successfully conquered.

Chapter 13:
Building a Successful Business

Building a successful esthetician career requires hard work, dedication to perfection, continuing education, and a solid business plan. Many skilled skin technicians have failed to reach their financial goals because of many business factors not taken into account. Analyzing the market is one of the first things you have to consider. You should ask yourself some questions, like is there any market opening for your service? How can you differentiate so you will not be beaten by competition? Do you have a means to open your own place, or will you go work as an employee?

The esthetician business is a competitive one, and you should not expect to succeed right away, but with a good business plan, good strategy in place, and your strong desire to continue your education and master your skills, you can provide distinctive quality of service and create a strong, profitable business.

If you are planning to open your own salon, you must be an educated and marketing-driven person, while developing a unique level of customer service techniques that will set your skin care place above the others in your area. Keeping yourself on top of skin care technology, new product development, and new techniques will help you to become a successful specialist and successful business owner. In this chapter, I am presenting the most important aspects of business planning and conducting in easy comprehendible way.

Business Plan and Start Up Cost

Firstly, to open a new skin care business, you need to take into consideration your financial possibilities in order to cover all start up costs. In other words, how much money you can afford to invest to purchase equipment, furniture, skin care product, advertisement, marketing materials, etc. Secondly, you need to develop strong business plan, including determination of your target market and effective methods of advertising. Can you purchase all the equipment and supplies you need immediately or have you given yourself room to grow? The planning stage is where you will need to project all start up costs, equipment, supplies, furnishing, education (courses, seminars, industry shows), advertisement, etc. Covering all your bases before you start will give you an idea of your total build out costs.

If you do not have big investment capital, you can have a choice to lease the expensive equipment. Before make a decision, you should investigate the advantages of leasing against purchasing. By leasing, you do not need come up with the huge start-up capital. There are lenders who offer longer-term leases with lower monthly payments compared to if you purchased the equipment. By leasing the equipment, you have a choice to try the machine and see if it is something that your clients can benefit from. Will you have many clients who can sign up for 10-12 session of treatment with this device? Will this equipment show results as it promises? For example, Oxygen Jet can cost somewhere around $3,000- $7,000. If you purchase it right away, you might end up losing money, because you do not know how many clients will sign up for the series of oxygen treatments. To reach beneficial results for the skin equipment like Oxygen Jet, microdermabrasion, LED, and radio frequency require numerous sessions, somewhere from 10 to 15 treatments.

Part of developing a business plan includes setting up your goals for weekly or monthly profit and calculating routine business expenses. Whether beginning as an employee, independent contractor, or salon owner, you have to determine how much you need to earn in order to cover your overhead and have descent profit. You will need to determine how much revenue the business will need to generate in order to cover your monthly overhead. You must factor in the overhead, such a rent, supplies, insurance, advertising, and other business expenses to determine your "net profit" on particular treatments. Assuming your overhead expenses are paid on a monthly basis, add all overhead and divide the number of working days per month. So your daily overhead amount has to be no more that 25% of you daily income. In other words, your daily income has to average about 75% of your "net" profit. But regular daily profit is an ideal situation and not always possible, especially if you just opened your business.

At first, you may do better to prorate your overhead expenses and your profit on a weekly basis. Do not judge your income by looking at just one day, because it will vary day-to-day. Look how much you made at the end of month and set up your goals. Let's say you want to have net profit of 4K per month. Write down your goal or always keep it in mind, and do not get discouraged if you have slow day or week. Judge you success by looking at your overall monthly profit and business progression.

Over the period of time, you can compare which months of the year are slower and which are the busiest. This will help you to organize your monthly expenses for the slow months, or possibly take a vacation in slow times. Then you can also analyze what services are on demand, what services are not very popular, and possibly promote unpopular businesses by offering small discounts, etc.

Choosing Business Structure, Business Location and Business Name

When it comes to the place of your business operation, you have two choices: You can buy or rent a small place and be a one-person business operator. Or you can rent the room from a salon owner/operator who will collect a flat monthly fee from you. You as an independent contractor must provide your own supplies, equipment, book your own appointments, and do your own sales taxes and so forth.

I know that many estheticians start their carrier working for big salons, earning their income by commission from their services. After they build solid clientele, they might consider opening their own business or becoming an independent contractor in the same salon or another one. Opening your own place often comes as the next logical step for those skin care professionals who have been successful. Owning your own shop implies a better quality of the services that you can offer, and this is also more attractive to your customers. Being a owner-operator, you will have financial benefits since all the profit that you make will go to you. It will allow expanding your services and increasing your potential even higher. But you are going to be day-to-day responsible for all aspects of business operation; scheduling your own appointments, paying your sales tax and income tax, bookkeeping, making financial decisions, ordering product, etc. All of this is in addition to providing treatments to your customers.

One of the first decisions that you have to make before you open your business is how the business should be structured. The basic legal forms of ownership for small businesses are Sole Proprietorship, Corporation, and Limited Liability Company (LLC). Most small salons start out as sole proprietorships. It is a business that is owned by one person who is normally active in running and managing the business.

After you choose your business structure, you need to pick your business location. Choosing a location for your skin care business or salon is one the most important decisions that you will make in the early stages of establishing. Obviously, you will want to locate it in an area that easy accessible, with plenty of traffic and parking. The surrounding area should be attractive, well lighted, and safe. It is preferable that there should be another business related to beauty or medical services nearby, as opposed to commercial areas, like industrial parks or regional airports.

When choosing a business name, you have to consider several important things; you want to choose a business name that is memorable, and it should be good for business promotion. First, you have to create name that your potential customers can easy to find in the phone book, directory, or online. It should contain easy spelling and relatively short words. When I was choosing the name for my business, one of my friends, who was a very experienced businessman, gave me suggestions to use the first word of the business starting with letter "A". This way salon will be always listed in the beginning of all listing for the beauty salon in the area where I lived. I named my business "Ambiance European Skin Care" and my salon was always listed first in the local yellow pages book. The name "Ambiance European Skin care" worked especially well since it had contained information of what services the business has been providing.

A winning business name has to be fairly short and easy to remember. It is also important for promotional purposes, since it should fit well on a business card and stand out on a sign. If you will consider having a website for your business, it will serve well as a domain name and will show up quickly in search.

No doubt, you will spend hours brainstorming for a business name that represents your services and will be both marketable and infused with personality. To help the creative process along, you might surf the Internet, browse the dictionary, read professional magazines, and bounce ideas off your friends and colleagues. But as you hunt for the perfect name, keep in mind all the advice that I gave to you when you are going to make the decision.

Business Marketing Tools

One of the main business marketing tools is design your own logo. The right logo, with the right characteristics, will boost your visibility and credibility. Your logo has to stand out from the crowd, try to create something unique that differentiates you from your competitors. Also your business logo has to contain the message about the distinguishing characteristics of your services. Your business cards, brochures, and business sign should include the logo of your business.

To design business cards, you need to keep in mind that it determines the perception of someone's first impression about you. Basically, it should hold the information about you and your place.

First, introduce yourself, e.g. include your business name, nature of your business, your name, and some of your credentials. For example, Durango Beauty Studio, Advanced Skin Therapy, Nancy Bronson, CIDSCO certified esthetician. You can also include your company logo or, if you do not have one, include your picture. If you notice, business cards with the picture of the business owner stand out the most.

Secondly, include contact information so that person can reach you. This means, include at least, if not all of, the following information: email address, website, URL (if you have one), phone numbers, and address. And lastly, get quality printing for your business cards. There are two main factors that determine the quality of the color, the printing job, and the quality of paper.

There are many websites that offer excellent quality printing, pre-designed business cards, and templates for different categories. And you can also design your own card and save it on file for re-ordering. I use a great, inexpensive online printing company, called Vista Print (www.vistaprint.com). Vista Print offers business cards, brochures, car magnets, address labels, etc. There is a very simple way to create your business tools at affordable prices.

A well- crafted sign can boost your business success by drawing more customers. Design your sign with a clear and short message. You do not want your sign to be cluttered with words and phrases. Rather, you want to put a short message that can be read quickly. For most people, take a glance to read the sign. Think of the message you want them to read during that time. If the message catches their attention, they will want to learn more. Sign with contrasting color has definite advantage over signs with similar colors. And try to avoid too many colors; I would say two contrasting colors might be the best choice. Place your sign in a visible spot of the building or put it above the building to make it easily seen. The sign of your business does not have to be a costly investment. You can design it yourself and order it with online companies who offer varieties of materials. The neon sign has advantages and disadvantages, so I do not recommend going with one. The only neon sign that you have to consider is the message sign like "Open", "Skin care", "Waxing", and more. They are eye-catching and deliver a clear message.

Bookkeeping and Accounting

Bookkeeping is often seen as chore that must be tolerated to stay in business. Some skin care professionals are even afraid to open their own business, because they do not know how to do bookkeeping and accounting. In reality, the bookkeeping can be very simple and easy if you organize it well with simple Bookkeeping Ledge or QuickBooks software. It may be somewhat time consuming, but once you learn how to do it; it might take only an extra hour per month to keep all your records. If you have your own place or you are self-contractor for a big salon or spa, it is more profitable to do your own books. Much software have a simple and easy way of letting you record your all start up expenses, your sales, and your monthly expenses for rent, telephone, insurance, supplies, etc.

When I first open my skin care business, I was doing my own bookkeeping, believing that I could save some money by doing accounting tasks myself. I did not have a computer, and, honestly speaking, I did not have computer skills back then. All my expenses, I kept record in a Monthly Bookkeeping Ledger, updating it once per month. I also kept all my receipts for tax purposes and kept record of all product sales and performed services in a separate book. At the end of each month, I was calculating the difference between gross profit, including services and product retail and how much I spent for the business maintenance. I did it just to see how my business was progressing and to know what time of year is the busiest time for company. However, for business tax preparation, I did hire an accounting service to help me properly file my tax returns.

In conclusion, if you are a single operator or independent contractor and do not have a computer, simply use the ledger books to handle your bookkeeping.

You need two basic "books":

1. A sales ledger to record details of all the sales that you make (retail product and the services).

In your sales ledger, you will enter all your services, including date, nature of the treatment, and charge and product that you sell. Retail product should be entered, including tax charge for your references when you need to pay sales tax to State and City. Usually, you have to pay the sales taxes quarterly or if you sales volume is very low, you can pay annually. Sales ledger must have the correct records of all of your income, where you list each source of income. It will include your charges for treatments, retail product, tips, and booth rentals fees. It depends on the structure of your business.

2. Purchases ledger ("simplified monthly bookkeeping record") to record details of all the purchases that you make for the business during the mouth. Also you have to record your expanses for rent, insurance, utility, telephone, sales tax, office supplies, etc.

All of these books can be found at office supply stores. You also need a Sales Receipt book that you can hand out receipt to your customers after the product sale.

Remember, even though you have reordered all your invoices and receipts, you still need to keep these "prime" documents as evidence for six years. Split them into sales and purchases and file them monthly. To help you find the original documents, you might want to consider numbering them and cross-referencing this number to your sales and purchase ledgers.

Keeping records can be very simple if you will do it on an every day basis. Do not pile up all you receipts and enter once per month; that can be somewhat overwhelming. Records for the sales order have to be done right after service or sales. This way, you will remember all your charges for which you perform service or sell the cosmetics. In a separate spreadsheet or "book", keep record of your inventory in accurate order, avoiding being overstocked or running short on your supplies for retail product

Also, it is necessarily to keep good records of all of your equipment and other valuable properties (office furniture, computer, and so forth) at your business. Because business assets wear out, you are allowed to write off (or depreciate) part of the cost of your assets over the period of time.

And lastly, you need to conduct service records that should contain the name, address, telephone, and email address of the client, date, and treatment performed. Product uses, recommendations, results, and other specific remarks. I can also recommend that you try to keep record of you client's birthday, since you can use it to send a treatment discount and so forth.

When you decide to add more employees to your salon, the bookkeeping may become somewhat complicated and time consuming. With simple application like QuickBooks, it appears easy and more accurate to keep your financial information. Using QuickBooks software allows you to track all of your inventory as well as sales. The program allows you to generate reports at any time so that you know where you stand financially.

If you own a big salon, I recommend that you hire an accountant to help with all records, payroll (if any), and filling tax returns. The accountant will have you nicely organized and detailed records when comes time to file tax return; this is far better that a huge jumble of receipts, scribbled notes, etc.

Pricing Your Services and Retail Product

Your business income will come from two sources: your service and retail products. The biggest part of you profit will generate from your services, and you have to make the right decisions when establishing a price list.

So, you need to take into consideration the economic situation in your area, competition level, how much your competitors charge for the same services, and what is your level of expertise in skin care field.

For example, highly educated and experienced estheticians can be confident to price her services quite higher than skin care services down the street. Remember, your credentials, as a specialist will be considered before the price of the treatment when it comes to choosing a skin care professional. Over the years, I have realized that majority of people who are looking for an esthetician considers better quality of service over lower price. However, setting prices too high can limit the number of people who can afford your treatment, and you will limit you profit potential.

Of course, the price the market will bear is very much dependent on the demographics of your service area. If you are in upscale area with larger homes occupied by people with more disposable income, you can price your services accordingly and can offer high-end skin care treatments. But if your surrounding community is populated with students or young working families, you can concentrate more on basic facial procedures and even offer some student discount treatments.

When setting your prices, you must consider other factors, like product and equipment cost, your overhead, and your competitors' pricing. Your overhead cost consists of all costs required to operate the business other than labor. This includes your mortgage or lease payment, utilities, accounting, and material cost. It is reasonable to estimate your overhead to be somewhat around 10% of the treatment cost.

Review your overhead expenses twice per year. It allows you to see which expenses have increased and which ones have remained the same. If you discovered that certain products have increased, try to replace this product with a less expensive one by doing your research. If you have noticed, my idea to keep overhead low is to use inexpensive "do-it-yourself" formulas that really work wonders and do not cost you a fortune. But, in cases when you purchased an expensive skin care system or equipment, you need consider increasing your prices for those services to make up the cost of your investment. Explain to your client the benefits of new treatment without being afraid to lose clients or revenue.

Be wise when you decided to invest in advanced skin care equipment, especially if you just open. It is great to offer varieties of treatments for your people, but remember that most people come for basic facials, like acne treatment or anti-aging moisturizing facials. Be excellent in those procedures and first purchase what you really need for basic skin care: facial bed, steamer, magnifying lamp, sanitizer, hot cabin, a Wood's lamp, high frequency, Galvanic, microdermabrasion machine. Other advanced skin care tools can be added later when you start generating some income keeping in mind that not all skin care equipment really does what it promises. Choose carefully and do your research. Refer to the **Chapter 14: "Advanced Skin Care Equipment"** where I am guiding you though varieties of advanced esthetic machinery and tools. The information will help you to make a right decision when it comes to purchasing devices that sufficiently treat skin problems.

I also want to mention the retail part of your business, which can be a very profitable if you choose a good advertising strategy. How many times you have passed opportunity to offer your product to the client? Do you advertise your product using eye-catching posters in your business place?

Introduce your product placing it in visible place. As I have mentioned, posters, brochures, and flyers are all good aids for retail part of business. There are several ways to develop and design business materials. Having them professionally designed and printed should be figured into your overhead expenses. There are many online printing companies that are offering high-quality printed marketing materials, promotional products, and marketing services, such as copywriting, design, websites, and postcard mailing. I can refer you to one of them that I have been using for years for all my business marketing needs: wwww.vistaprint.com. This company offers all marketing tools for an inexpensive cost.

Educate your customer about your product features and benefits while doing their treatment. It is a vital part of success is to suggest and sell home care products to your clients.

Do not push your product to the clients if they are satisfied with the products that they are using at home. However, do offer suggestions

Do not try overwhelming your customers with multi-step home care routine. Remember, most people are more receptive to the basic steps for skin care.

Carry private label product to insure that nobody in your area has the same product. The Ray Lab, Inc offers private labels product as well as many another skin care companies. Having your company name on quality product will protect your profit and will bond your relationship with the customers.

Advertising Your Business

When you decided to start advertising your business, you have to keep in mind that the average advertising cost should not exceed 3-5% of your gross income. This percentage should be figured into your overhead, while allowing 8% for your rent, 6-8% for your supplies, 7% for all utilities and telephone, 5-6% for all taxes, and 2% for insurance. Your bookkeeping or accounting expenses should be no more than 2%, and this is in case you hire an accountant. If you are an independent contractor or a one-person business operator, the best idea is to do books and tax preparation by yourself, using special software or bookkeeping ledgers.

Before you spend money on a newspaper advertisement that will reach the entire city or town that you live in, you must first to decide on an advertising budget and in which newspaper your ad will be most effective. A newspaper ad can run from one day to five, sometimes including the weekend, and it is very expensive. I have found the majority of newspapers are more widely read on Wednesday and Friday, than any other day of the week. Planning to run your ad on one of these days will give it more visibility. I also found that it is more effective to run your ad in the area business magazine versa the weekly newspaper, because the majority of people keep magazines for several weeks or months, especially if it features "dollars off" for first clients. This type of advertisement worked very well for me when I first opened my business. I would go with this one before the newspaper advertisement.

For introducing your new business to your area, you can also use local "mail-in coupons" for your company offering special discounts for first time clients. The "mail-in" usually reaches all people living in your area, and the majority of them use this coupon for their service needs.

Mailing directly to existing customers is a good idea as well in order to increase their visits. Special events promotion or "reminder" postcard can be announced by mailing it to you clients. For example, you can put it like this: "It has been 2 months since your last facial treatment" or something like that.

In addition, I discovered another way to keep in touch with your existing clients: emailing them any business newsletter or announcement with the promotion. It is easy and free for you and works very efficiently.
It is not a secret that now-a-days more people communicate by email, and it does not have to cost you a penny.

One of the best, least expensive and free forms of advertising is word of mouth. The client should leave your place feeling great herself or himself and confident in your ability and knowledge. One satisfied client could tell ten of her or his friends. Of those ten, three will call to schedule an appointment with you, and one will remain loyal to you. The same it works the other way around, so be consistent with your services.

To jump-start your business, you have to advertise your business in any possible way. You can hand out your business card to restaurant owners, hotels, sport clubs, holistic centers, and so forth. I always carry my business cards and samples of my product with me wherever I go. I know I could meet my client with the friend, or meet someone in the bank or grocery store who might be interested in my trade. So be prepared and always have your advertising "tools" with you.

In addition, in the beginning of my esthetician carrier, I conducted several skin care educational seminars in establishments like banks, real estate agencies, high schools, and more. You can use your own intuition to see who can be interested in skin care seminar. For instance, acne skin care seminar can evoke interest among high school teenagers. Many of them are not aware how to properly take care of their skin during puberty period that can be very problematic. Offer special discount for school students, and stay on top of teens needs.

Another "free" form of advertising is to associate your business with the local dermatologist that is knowledgeable in skin diseases and disorders. Write them a letter offering them cooperation in exchanging referrals for clients in need of specialized services. Include your business cards and brochures and invite them to visit your skin care place, offering a free treatment for the dermatologist.

If your business is located close to a hotel or motel ask the manager permission to leave your brochures at the front desk in case their guests inquire about skin care services. You might consider offering discount coupons to the hotel staff for their referrals, or to the guests themselves. You can try the same approach with other businesses in your area.

Flyers with some special deals also can be a free advertising, especially for such services like waxing or eyelash tint. This is one is my least favorite methods of advertisement, but I know few of my colleagues for whom this approach has worked very well.

In conclusion, new customers just do not walk into your place every day. Advertising your business requires careful planning and effective strategies. Aside from traditional ways of advertisement - newspaper, radio, and yellow pages - there are other ways to get prospective customers through the doors of your business that are sometimes less costly and more effective. Use your creativity and strong effort, and it will generate you more clients and, ultimately, more money.

CHAPTER 14:
ADVANCED SKIN CARE TECHNOLOGY

Once a year, I attend the International Esthetician conference because I want to be on top of new technology in the skin care industry. It seems very overwhelming how many new skin care devices and tools are offered by manufacturers around the world. All of them promise great results for treating specific skin conditions, like fine lines, hyper pigmentation, acne, rosacea, broken capillaries, sagging, scarring, unwanted hair, and more. You can easily spend a fairly large amount of money to purchase these skin care tools.

When I first began my business, I was like most skin care professionals, and I wanted to perform the most advanced skin care treatments. And so, I simply purchased nearly all of them: Microdermabrasion, LED light therapy, low-level laser, ultrasonic massager, micro current stimulation, infrared blanket, oxygen jet and Radio Frequency. Adding them to my services, I was able to test all of them during a sufficient amount of time. Finally, I have realized that not every one of them provides beneficial results to the skin.

A variety of new technology and esthetic equipment can be used to soften fine lines, even out skin tone, reduce acne scars, and increase skin elasticity. All of these technologies claim to work by stimulating natural collagen production of the skin. In this chapter, I want to help estheticians make proper decisions on their purchase when they decide to add new skin care equipment to their practice.

Microdermabrasion Equipment

This equipment is one of the most successful esthetic tools that have been introduced about decade ago and is still now-a-days widely used by estheticians. I am big fan of microdermabrasion techniques, and it has become very popular among all my clients, because it provides excellent results. My protocol of microdermabrasion procedure is somewhat different than has been offered by the majority esthetic courses. Please, refer to the **Chapter 8: "Microdermabrasion**

and Chemical peels" for the detailed description of the microdermabrasion treatment.

Once again, I want to mention, that there are two types of microdermabrasion equipment available on market; diamond tip (crystals free) and crystal microdermabrasion. Both of those machineries perform in a similar manner but have disadvantages and advantages relative each other. Do your research before you decide to purchase one or the other, and choose what is more suitable for you. I am not going to describe all the details here. But, remember, one of the criteria of choosing a manufacturer who you are going to purchase the equipment from is what kind of educational support they provide with the purchase.

Ultrasound Massager

This is one of my favorite treatment enhancing tools. The ultrasound technology has been used for physical therapy for years, and just recently, it was introduced to esthetic treatments. Wide therapeutic use is safe and easy to use, and providing great results has made ultrasonic instruments very popular among skin care professionals.

What are ultrasound waves? The term "ultrasonic" applies to sound and refers to anything above the frequencies of audible sound. In other words, ultrasonic sound waves are at a frequency of more than 20,000HZ and are not heard by the human ear. For skin care, most machines are created at 1MHz with continuous and pulsed frequencies. Produced by ultrasonic devices, high frequency waves have tremendous therapeutic effect on human skin by delivering three main benefits: micro-massage (vibration), heating effect, and cavitations (deep product penetration).

The ultrasound waves have the ability penetrate up to 2" deep into skin and facilitate skin-rejuvenating processes by improving cell metabolism. It can promote collagen production; therefore increase skin elasticity and firmness. Ultrasound vibration improves blood and lymph circulation that delivers an anti-inflammatory effect for skin problems, like acne or rosacea. Warming action is one of the most important therapeutic factors of ultrasound skin care tool since it produces internal heat that also increases blood flow and speeds up the healing processes.

In my opinion, ultrasound devices are one of the most superior aids for delivering skin care product into skin. The cavitation action of ultrasound waves provides maximum absorption of the cosmetic product, therefore giving skin the most benefits from facial creams, serums, and lotions. The Galvanic method also promotes skin product penetration, but in some cases, I prefer the ultrasound massager since you can use any skin care product, and you do not have to think about product polarity. In contrary, Galvanic method can be used for products that are positively or negatively ionized. I will describe Galvanic treatment in detail further in this chapter.

The Benefits of an Ultrasound Massager:

- Increases skin elasticity, and helps to reduce fine lines
- Enhances skin product absorption, and therefore, promotes nutrients and moisture delivery
- Diminishes unwanted pigmentation by destroying melanin
- Provides anti-inflammatory action by increasing blood circulation.

Based on the above information, estheticians can use an ultrasonic device for anti-aging, post microdermabrasion, mild acne, and rosacea treatments.

Ultrasonic Scrubber

This is the newest application of ultrasound technology. The device has one stainless steel panel that produces ultrasound waves. When it contacts the surface of the skin, it glides over and removes dead cells, comedones, and another skin's impurities. This tool is very helpful for extraction. I use it before the manual extraction with the steam or right after steaming the face. It complements microdermabrasion and provides more efficient exfoliation. High frequency of the device can soften epidermis; helps remove excessive oil, cleans plugged pores, and brightens up pigment spots. The result is a remarkable and cleaning effect that is guaranteed. This process is totally non-invasive and can be used for sensitive skin as well. But never use the ultrasonic scrubber on inflamed skin, such as acute severe acne skin condition.

Galvanic Device

This is a very valuable tool for skin care treatments. It is a fairly old technique and has been used in Europe for more than four decades. It has been utilized to treat moderate and severe acne skin inflammation, hyper pigmentation, and skin rejuvenation.

Galvanic device produces continuous current that dissociate molecules on positive and negative ions in order to move them to positive and negative electrodes. The positive ions begin to accumulate on the contact of the active or negatively charged electrode (cathode) and the negative ions drawn toward the inactive (silent), positively charged electrode (anode). The produced effect is called ionization. The purpose of ionization is to facilitate penetration of cosmetic products into skin. The skin products, like serums, vitamin solutions, antibacterial ointments, and dis-incrustation solutions must have known polarity to use them for facial treatments. If the product has positive polarity, the active electrode is attached to positive pole (+) of the galvanic device and the inactive electrode to the negative pole (-) of the device. If the treatment product is negative (-), the electrodes are connected in an opposite manner. Do not use galvanic device if a person has dermatitis, eczema, or rosacea, and do not use it for pregnant women as well.

The device is equipped with metal tips that look like a roller or flat metal plate. The person who operates the equipment is an active electrode, and polarity has to be adjusted according to the polarity of skin care product. The inactive electrode is the metal or rubber plate that has to be held in a client's hand. For better current conduction, the inactive electrode has to be covered with gauze, saturated with salty water. The active electrode has to be covered with fabric, saturated with the skin care product and applied on treated areas (face or neck). Slowly moving the electrode around on the treated spot, the esthetician needs to make sure that the active electrodes always stay attached to the skin. The duration of the procedure usually lasts for 10 min. For the best result, galvanic treatment should be performed right after extraction (acne facial). For the acne treatment, the esthetician should use disincrustation solution that helps to soften sebum and open the pores. The easiest way to prepare disincrustation solution is to use baking soda and distilled water. Use 1 tsp of baking soda and 2 ounces distilled water.

There are several substances that can be used for galvanic facial treatments to enhance the skin care therapy.

Aloe gel 1-2%   (-) polarity.

Can used do for healing and calming purposes on oily or irritated skin

Hyaluronic acid 2%   (+) polarity

Effective for deep moisturizing or anti-aging treatments (microdermabrasion or European facial)

Ichthammol 20% ointment   (-) polarity

Contains: Petrolatum, ichthammol, anhydrous lanolin and light mineral oil.

Treatment with ichthammol provides great results for cystic acne treatments in order to diminish inflamed nodules, skin abscesses, and posy cists.

Vitamin C (ascorbic acid 2-5%)   (-) polarity

Galvanic treatment provides deep penetration of Vitamin C for post-microdermabrasion step.

H202 (Hydrogen peroxide) 5-10% (-) polarity

10 min of galvanic procedure provides deep bleaching effect and can be used or hyper pigmentation treatments.

Some serums designed by professional skin care lines provide great results if delivered by means of galvanic procedure. All you have to know is the polarity of product for it to be delivered to the skin. In most times, polarity is positive, but you have to contact the manufacturer of the product for the information.

The Benefits of Galvanic Treatments:

- Provides deep product delivery into skin dermal layer where product accumulates
- Provides extended realization of product for extended benefits
- Provides ability to deliver product directly to treated area
- Delivery of product is safe and completely pain free

High Frequency

For your knowledge, high frequency technology is not a very new. Hungarian Scientist Nikola Tesla first developed high frequency current in the late 1800's. French physicist D'Arsonval did more research in this discovery and introduced the use of high frequency currents to treat diseases of the skin and mucous membranes. The current is now known as the D'Arsonval high frequency current and that's how this technology is referred to in Europe.

By the 1970's or even earlier, European spas and salons discovered the cosmetic and healing benefits of high frequency electrical stimulation, and by 1980, the technology became widely used in North American.

The safe, non-invasive therapy was quickly found to be very beneficial in the treatment of many skin conditions, ranging from acne to wrinkles. Many estheticians use the power of high frequency technology on their clients, due to its ability to kick-start the skin rejuvenation process. The safe and gentle oscillating, oxygenating power of high frequency electrical current has been shown to enhance blood circulation, increase collagen and elastin production, eliminate toxins and acne-causing bacteria, encourage lymphatic drainage, exfoliate dead skin cells, and assist with skin care product absorption.

The electrodes for the high frequency are made of glass, and their shapes will vary depending on which part of the body is going to be treated. All treatments given with high frequency should start with a mild current, and gradually increase to the required strength. The length of the treatment depends upon the condition to be treated. For a general facial treatment, approximately three to five minutes should be allowed.

When applied to the surface of the skin or scalp, a mild high frequency electrical current passes through the neon or argon gas-filled glass electrode, causing it to light up with a calming orange-red or violet purple glow. The device provides painless tingling sensation that facilitates blood circulation in the dermal layer of the skin. High frequency current produces molecules of ozone that deliver oxygen to the skin. Ozone is a gas that has antibacterial properties and is successfully used for acne treatments. Use a "mushroom" shaped glass electrode, massaging congested skin areas for 5-8 min. The high frequency massage is a great addition for acne or oily skin treatments since it helps to close pores after extraction, regulating skin's oil production and disinfecting the skin.

The device is indicated for numerous of skin problems like acne, seborrhea, dermatitis, eczema, psoriasis, dull, lack of tone, and oily skin. Lately, the method has been successfully used as anti-aging aid to treat wrinkles and fine lines. But to see obvious results, it is required that you have many treatments that are more suitable for home use.

The Benefits of High Frequency Treatments:

- Stimulates blood and lymph circulation
- Provides cell oxygenation
- Provides better product absorption
- Increases cells metabolism
- Provides antibacterial properties

High frequency facial treatments are considered to be a safe and gentle approach to skin rejuvenation treatment; however, the following precautions should be taken: Do not use high frequency on skin with dilated and broken capillaries, known as couperose skin condition. Avoid using it on clients who suffer with rosacea and never use it to treat cystic acne with numerous nosy nodules on the skin, since it can spread bacteria all over the face. Avoid using AHA, Glycolic, or another peel with the system.

Micro-Current Therapy

This claims to provide outstanding results for face lifts, while tone the muscle and firms the skin. Micro-current is a modality providing electric current in millionths of an ampere. Used since the 1940s as a physical therapy treatment, it has the ability to relieve pain, increase tissue healing and regeneration, increase protein synthesis, stimulate lymphatic flow, and relieve myofascial trigger points. Because micro-current flows at one million of an ampere, it is delivered on the same scale as the current that the human body produces on its own in each cell. The human body cannot feel such small electrical currents; therefore, the micro-current procedure is completely safe and painless. A micro-current device sends safe impulses to the facial muscles to tighten, tone, and firm. It not only helps muscles to relax, but it also helps weak muscles regain strength, thus increasing its volume and firmness. Micro-current facelift procedure takes approximately one hour to complete and requires no anesthesia, no recovery time, no down time from work, and has no irritating side effects. An esthetician uses a two-pronged, cotton-tipped instrument to gently deliver electrical stimulation to the muscles and tissues of the face and neck. To achieve the ultimate benefits of a micro current facelift, approximately twelve sessions are recommended. Most clients need about 10 treatments to achieve a look that shaves off 7-10 years or more. Clients with severe neck sagging, deep wrinkles, or distinguished "crow's feet" may need up to 15 sessions a week apart. Those who are on a short timeline or those who desire extra work on trouble areas may be treated twice per week. Once treatment sessions are complete, the routine maintenance of one treatment per month is recommended.

The Benefits of Micro-Current Treatment:

- Improves muscle tone in the face and neck
- Lifts jowls and eyebrows
- Diminishes and softens fine lines and wrinkles
- Increases facial circulation, lymphatic drainage, and product penetration
- Exfoliates the skin
- Minimizes sun damage and unwanted pigmentation

The majority of skin care professionals working with micro-current became amazed with the results for some clients and frustrated with the results for others. While I was doing my own research testing the micro-current device, I have been noticed the same thing; while it produces results for one person it does not affect another. There is no explanation for this phenomenon, but I assume it has to do with the individual response to the micro-current. Besides if it did produce certain visible result of face lift, the effect could last only for several months or less, so the repetition of the session was required to maintain the benefits of the treatment.

Electro Stimulating Devices

Electro-stimulating devices are devices that use electronic muscle stimulation to provide visible improvement for saggy skin around the mouth, cheeks, chin, and jaws area. The systems produce continuous pulses of micro-current that contacts and releases the muscles of the face simulating physical exercise. Unfortunately, facial group muscles are not giving as much attention as other muscles of the body, and as we got older, they tend to atrophy and provide a droopy look.

Electronic Muscle Stimulation

This is an advanced technique, used worldwide, for toning, reshaping, and firming different groups of muscles of the body. An electronic muscle stimulator uses electrical signals to tense and release muscles, through the employment of small electrodes on either side of the muscle area. By placing the pair of pads on a particular muscle group, muscles respond to the impulses that are generated by contracting and relaxing rhythmically as instructed by a technician through the unit. An electrical current mimics brain's instructions to muscles and smoothly contracts and relaxes each muscle, exercising, toning, and revitalizing it.

There are many models of the EMS devices available on market for home and salon use. They all claim permanent improvement after a significantly long period of use. The result usually can be seen within 3-4 weeks of daily use. That indicates that using this technology for salon treatments probably is not going to be as effective as someone who will use it at home every day.

Using the EMS for facial muscles is a relatively new technology and can be unsafe if the device is not properly used or device itself came from an unknown manufacturer from Asia. It is very important that these devices were properly designed; manufactured, and labeled with clear and complete instructions for use. The companies must be able to demonstrate that these devices are safe and effective as similar devices that are legally marketed. The only one EMS device that has been approved by FDA is Slendertone Flex, marketed by BMR NeuroTech, Inc. At this time, the FDA is not aware of scientific information to support many of the promotional claims being made for numerous devices being widely promoted on television, infomercials, newspapers, and magazines. Recently, the FDA has received reports of shocks, burns, bruising, skin irritation, and pain associated with the use of some of these devices. There have been a few recent reports of interference with implanted devices, such as pacemakers. Estheticians have to always ask their clients about any health issue before they consider performing any treatment related to electric current application.

I do not use any EMS devices in my business due to unrealistic treatment conditions. As I have mentioned before, it can be very costly and time consuming for the person to see the desirable result, since the treatment has to be done almost every day. But some of my client have used the equipment at home on a regular basis and reported some improvement. However, several people experienced mixed results with EMS devices as some improvement with negative results on the eye area that create some swelling and puffiness. Skin around the eye is very delicate and any aggressive stimulation can cause broken capillaries or tissue damage. My recommendation would be, if you want to try this product, avoid using it around the eyes.

Oxygen Therapies

For the beauty industry, these revolve around the use of medical grade oxygen as a delivery mechanism for active ingredients in to the skin. Oxygen Jet system contain oxygen concentrator that produces 95% oxygen and has an airbrush that sprays nutrients on the client's face and mask connected to oxygen concentrator to provide "oxygen bath". The airbrush attachment is designed to spray oxygen with cosmetic nutrients on specific areas of the face or body. With 0.3mm nozzle size, the airbrush disperses liquid into tiny drops and sprays on the skin. "Oxygen bath" is a plastic mask that is connected with oxygen concentrator by a plastic tube and evenly delivers 95% oxygen to the skin.

Oxygen Jet

This is the system that performs so-called "oxygen facials". It claims to deliver serums composed of antioxidants, amino acids, and vitamins to the skin through oxygen to hydrate and nourish aging skin. The key function of oxygen here is theorised to be an increased absorption of the active ingredients. Similar to what would be experienced with ionophoresis (Galvanic treatment). The treatments are supposed to leave skin younger and plumped up with a visible firming effect.

While many skin care professionals see some benefits from high-pressure oxygen facial others are taking a more skeptical approach to this procedure. Oxygen facials are another modality that is increasing in popularity, but also raising a number of questions about effectiveness and credibility due to both the lack of scientific evidence and the growing awareness of the link between oxygen and free radical damage.

I did my own research on how effective the oxygen facial is and how long the results last. I did notice that skin looks plumed and radiant after using oxygen spray with hyaluronic acid serum or multivitamin solution. But results were not permanent even after series of 10 or 12 treatments. The pluming effect lasted basically a few days the most. When I was combining oxygen-infused treatments with microdermabrasions, the result was long lasting and, in most cases, permanent. So I was not really sure if high-pressure injections with the oxygen were enhancing microdermabrasion since microdermabrasion itself produces permanent skin improvement. But the one skin benefit that I can mention for sure, the oxygen spray or oxygen bath is a very cooling and soothing addition to the post -microdermabrasion step of facials. It helps to accelerate the healing process after any hash, abrasive treatment, like microdermabrasion or chemical peels. I have also noticed that oxygen can give some relief for acne problems since oxygen provides antibacterial properties, but it has to be used along with traditional acne facial steps.

In conclusion, the oxygen has limited benefits and have no value rather than as an addition to serious skin treatments. The equipment is costly and can run somewhere between $3000 and $10,000. If you are seriously considering investing in this device, do not expect to get your money back soon.

Photo Facials or Skin Light Therapy

Skin therapy using Low Level Laser, LED therapy (light emitting diode), intensive light therapy (IPL), or RF (radio frequency) techniques is becoming increasingly popular since more people are looking for non-invasive, no down time techniques to obtain younger looking skin, get rid of unwanted pigmentation, or eliminate visible blood vessels. Recently developed photo rejuvenation devices like LED, Low-level laser and IPL address are all skin photo-aging elements, which include pigment spots, enlarged pores, telangiectasia, and fine lines. All these advanced treatments utilize light and heat energy that has different wavelengths. These are lasers and IPL sources emitting a visible wavelength that convert into heat, resulting in coagulation of visible capillaries, moderate burn of epidermis, and mild heating of dermis. The thermal action to the epidermis helps to destroy build up of melanin. On the other hand, the thermal "injury" to dermal layer of skin leads to activation and synthesis of new collagen fiber. Therefore, the skin responds with significant improvement in texture and color.

Medical professionals (plastic surgeons, dermatologists, etc.) use different models of Laser to treat skin problems. Types of lasers like the Pearl laser, YAG laser, and CO2 resurfacing can erase years from the face and dramatically improve aging skin. Although highly effective, there are the thermal discomfort considerations that some clients will not be prepared to accept hot lasers; the kind used by health professionals in the treatment of skin resurfacing and tattoo removal. The high-energy devices that cause heat damage to the skin have to be performed under local or even general anesthesia and require some time to recover.

Fractional Resurfacing

This offers a less invasive alternative to traditional laser resurfacing. It allows for skin improvements with minimal risk and little downtime, because each treatment creates thousand of microscopic wounds, while leaving the surrounding skin intact. Over a series of office visits, the client notices significant improvement in skin texture, diminishing fine lines, and skin unwanted pigmentation.

With so many types of laser treatments, people who want to improve their skin condition are often confused. The best advice is to find a physician that is well versed in lasers and has experience, using multiple technologies so that they can advise their clients of the best solution for their concerns.

IPL (Intense Pulse Light) Treatment

This works by employing a broad spectrum of light energy in a range of wavelengths. It is based on emitting high intensity pulses of light (*not* lasers) to penetrate the skin and rid it of various skin problems. There are different machines for different levels or types of penetration. It is also known as *IPL Photorejuvenation*.

IPL treatment destroys bothersome pigment in the skin, while simultaneously stimulating collagen production. The treatment helps to get rid of sun-damage, including age spots, broken capillaries, and fine lines. Procedures usually take only 30 minutes, and the person can return back to work or daily activities. IPL devices are easy to operate and relatively safe to use. Therefore, they are mostly preferred for esthetic treatments; however, in order to perform the treatments, estheticians have to work under the supervision of a medical professional.

The new term "paramedical esthetician" is not an unusual thing any longer and now-a-days many beauticians want to expand their knowledge in dermatological and plastic procedures. Paramedical Estheticians work with plastic surgeons and dermatologists in pre-and postoperative skin care. Under the guidance of a licensed health care provider, they can perform skin treatments like IPL and laser hair removal.

A cool laser is an esthetic device that can be a safe alternative to medical lasers. Cool lasers are sometimes called low-level lasers or low-level light therapy devices. This type of laser doesn't damage tissue, and it is safe to use for salon treatments.

It works by passing a beam of light through the skin to reach cells below the skin surface and stimulate natural healing processes into dermal level of skin. Energy produced by cool lasers facilitates the production of collagen and ATP (the energy source needed for cellular functions), promote blood circulation, and boost the release of growth factors and the removal of waste products from cells. Low-level lasers (LLL) produce a beam of light that has a specific wavelength and frequency, and it does not generate perceivable heat. Therefore, LLL treatments are painless, and patients experience no warmth or burning as a result of the medical laser.

LLT emits from 650 to 890 nm light wavelength, which is considered the most beneficial for skin rejuvenation processes. While some patients get immediate results, in mostly cases, it requires 6-12 treatments to see permanent results. The benefits are smooth and youthful looking skin. The LL lasers are a useful tool for esthetic treatments and can be used alone or as an addition to microdermabrasion and any rejuvenation procedures.

LED Skin treatments are one of the hottest facial rejuvenation treatments that offer totally natural, non-ablative method for skin improvements. LED Skin Rejuvenation is the interaction of light, delivered through Light Emitting Diodes (LED), to activate cell receptors, causing them to produce collagen molecules. It uses low intensity light-emitting diodes (LEDs) in a process similar to photosynthesis in which plants use chlorophyll to convert sunlight into cellular building blocks.

Yellow LEDs are used for photo-rejuvenation. It helps to smooth out fine lines and increase skin elasticity. Blue LEDs are used to improve acne skin condition. LED devices that employ blue light help to destroy bacteria that cause breakouts in the first place, and it also help to inhibit sebum production by sebaceous glands. Some LED facial devices contain blue and red light combined that provides antibacterial properties and reduces inflammation.

Red LEDs produce the same light frequencies as lasers but without the intense heat and tissue damage. Red LED skin treatments help to improve rosacea, remove skin blemishes, diminish hyperpigmentation, improve overall skin tone and texture, and decrease fine lines and wrinkles. Some LED devices emit a purple light that is usually weaker than red light. It can be used for lymph drainage facial massage to facilitate toxins removing from the head area or for anti-aging purposes as well.

Typically, treatments are spread over several months. The number of treatments and the treatment times will vary depending on the problem and the size of the area being treated. Since the results are progressive, clients will notice more correction with each treatment. Since the skin continues to age, maintenance procedures will be required. I usually recommend eight to ten weekly treatments, and for maintenance, one treatment per month is required. The recommended duration of LED skin treatments is 30 minutes, and it can be used alone or in conjunction with any anti-aging or anti-acne treatments. Maintenance treatments are recommended every 30-60 days.

While using the LED device, the technician has to be aware of some safety requirements. The technician has to avoid pointing the light beam directly into eyes of the client. It has been suggested that client's keep their eyes closed during the procedure. When work on the neck area, avoid over stimulation of thyroid glands.

For LED facial procedures, estheticians have included all the steps of a regular facial, including cleansing, exfoliation, extraction (for acne treatment), and nourishing or acne mask application at the end. Avoid using aggressive products (chemical peels) along with LED. Try to address more nourishing or moisturizing products for anti-aging treatments and acne products for acne facials. Since the LED can assist in hyperpigmentation treatment, the device can be used in conjunction with microdermabrasion treatment to diminish skin discoloration.

Radio Frequency

The radio frequency (RF) utilizes 10MHz/S electric waves, which can permeate the epidermis to take effect on the underlying tissues. The theory is that carefully controlled RF can be used for heating to contract deep dermal tissue without superficial heat injury. The technology is based on the principal of radio frequency electric waves that penetrate into the dermal layer of skin and gently heats collagen fibers, causing its coagulation. When deep collagen tissue is heated up to 45–60, it will naturally produce instant shrinking that stimulates production of new collagen molecules to make up created space. Over time, new and remodeled collagen is produced to further tighten the skin, resulting in healthier, smoother skin and a more youthful appearance. Creating heat in the epidermal layer is interpreted as an injury by the body and in response; the body produces more white cells, fibroblasts, and new collagen molecules. Since high heat causes immediate contraction of the fibers and collagen tissues, followed by new collagen production and recombination; hence, the desirable effects of skin-tightening, wrinkle-removal, and figure shaping, etc.

There are two types of RF devices that have been used by medical professionals to treat aging skin: monopolar and biopolar RF. Both monopolar and bipolar RF are used for tissue tightening. The main difference between these 2 categories lies in the configuration of the electrodes applied to the skin, with important repercussions on how the energy is conveyed into the skin itself and into the underlying tissues. Monopolar RF heats tissue in the treated area rather deeply (usually up to 20 mm), and thus, it affects both the skin and subcutaneous fat. Bipolar RF heats the tissue in the treated area less deeply (usually up to 2-4 mm) and, thus, primarily affects the skin.

Monopolar (also called Unipolar)

Monopolar, or unipolar, refers to a device having one pole or electrode. With monopolar delivery, the current from the RF device flows from a single electrode (headpiece) and meets maximum resistance in the area around the tip of the headpiece, where heat is occurring. Grounding pad should be attached to the patient's lower back or abdomen to provide a low resistance path and complete electrical circuit.

Numerous reports of a monopolar radio frequency (RF) device have indicated that this non-surgical option for reducing skin laxity with little or no downtime may be effective to address sagging of facial skin.

An example of a monopolar RF device used for facial rejuvenation and available in the USA is the ThermaCool by Thermage. In contrast to traditional ablative resurfacing techniques, the ThermaCool System (ThermaCool System, Thermage, Inc., Hayward, California) protects the skin surface from injury while selectively heating the underlying dermis. Preservation of epidermal integrity minimizes recovery and the risk of complications. The patient will experience a brief, deep heating sensation as the RF energy is delivered to the skin and underlying tissues. This deep heating sensation is an indication that dermal collagen is reaching effective temperatures for tightening. The physician controls the amount of energy delivered to balance procedural comfort with maximum results. Prior to treatment, an anesthetic cream may be applied to enhance the comfort.

Recently published studies conducted by Thermage show that measurable tightening improvements appear gradually over 2 to 6 months after a single treatment session. However, many patients have reported seeing an earlier response. The results vary from individual to individual and depend on a number of different factors, including age, the area treated, the amount of laxity in the skin, and how well a patient's skin responds.

Most people return to their regular activities immediately following the Thermage procedure. Some people experience mild redness (like a sunburn), but it usually disappears quickly. No special care is needed after treatment unless otherwise instructed by your physician.

Biopolar

Biopolar refers to a device having two poles or electrodes. The current passes between two identical electrodes located a short distance apart from each other. The depth reached by the current is equal to approximately half the distance separating the two electrodes. Bipolar systems, thus, ensure a better-controlled distribution of energy, and the patients treated with these devices tolerate the session with ease. Compared to the monopolar configuration, however, the depth of penetration of the current is less, and for this reason, it is difficult for it to reach the deep dermis and subcutaneous tissues.

The effects of both modalities are somewhat complementary, because they deliver energy in different patterns and to different depths. Combining monopolar and bipolar RF allows the reduction of the required intensity of each, and thus minimize side effects and possibly increase effectiveness (as compared to each type of radio frequency used alone). The combination of monopolar and bipolar radio frequency has been used for skin tightening, facial contouring, body sculpting, and cellulite reduction.

In conclusion, the RF devices proved to be effective, noninvasive, and easy to use. The improvement in the treated areas is progressive and continues to be apparent several months after the last session. The duration of the results achieved still remains to be accurately determined.

The Benefits of RF Applications:

- Provides skin-firming effects
- Improves skin elasticity
- Facilitates blood flow and lymph circulation
- Reduces skin inflammation
- Reduces fat tissue and diminishes cellulite
- Breast tissue tightening and lifting

RF energy has been used extensively in medicine over the past century to generate focused heat to cut and to coagulate tissue during surgery. For the past decade, RF technology was introduced to skin care industry to successfully to treat age-related skin problems. Up till now, this procedure has been performed in medical professional offices by plastic surgeons or trained dermatologists. In recent years, some medical esthetic programs are offering advanced training to operate with this high technology skin care equipment. The qualified licensed esthetician or cosmetologist can learn how to operate with varieties of medical esthetic modalities, like microdermabrasion, ultrasound, LED, IPL,

Laser, and Radio Frequency equipment. Upon completion of training program, they will be able to provide the treatments by themselves, alone, or under supervision of medical professionals, depending on the state board requirement of their current residency.

I hope this chapter will help you to make the right decision when it comes to choosing what esthetic device to add to your existing or new business. Do you own research to find a distributor or manufacturer that provides outstanding support for their customers, i.e. extended warranty, educational classes, parts supply, repairmen, etc.

A FINAL NOTE

I believe that the materials presented in my book will be a valuable asset for any skin care professional and can be marketed as an educational manual to the graduate beauty schools students. I believe that there is no available information on the details of European techniques that exist in the current market. I have also found that most of the available manuals are excessively expensive, and they don't offer practical techniques based on personal experience.

The only major competition is an esthetician manual by Milady's that represents excellent educational manual for estheticians students, but again, it does not contain practical information on every aspect of skin care business as well as European skin care techniques and detailed treatments protocols.

Thus, I know that many skin care professionals are looking for a compact and affordable manual that contains detailed skin care protocols. The techniques presented are traditional and holistic, but most importantly, they have been used successfully for generations. They have been refined over time, and with them, you can consistently achieve outstanding results in esthetic career.

BOOK REFERENCES AND RESOURCES

Hampton, Aubrey. 1987. Natural Organic Hair and Skin Care: Including A to Z Guide to Natural and Synthetic Chemicals in Cosmetics. *Organic Press*. 4419 N. Manhattan Ave., Tampa, FL 33614.

Balch, Phyllis A. and James. 2000. Prescription for Nutritional Healing. Third Edition. A Practical A-to- Z Reference to Drug-Free Remedies Using Vitamins, Minerals, Herbs & Food Supplements. Penguin Putnam Inc. 375 Hudson Street, New York, NY 10014. www.penguinputnam.com.

Page, Linda Rector, N.D; Ph.D. 1990. Healthy Healing: An Alternative Healing Reference. New Revised Expanded 8th Edition. Printed by Griffin Printing.

Begoun, Paula. 2008. Don't Go to the Cosmetics Counter Without Me. 7th Edition. Beginning Press, Washington 98057. www.Beautypedia.com

Glykhenkij, B.T. MD, Ph.D. of medical sciences. 1989. Manual of medical cosmetology. "Zdorovje". Kiev, USSR.

Tsisnetska A.V., S.Z. Kotuk. Modern Technology, Esthetic Procedures, Physiotherapy in Dermatology and Cosmetology.

Lviv State Medical University named after Danilo Halitsky. Lviv. 2008

Klimishina C.O., Tsisnetska A.V., Pachkevich L.V. Pharmaceutical Cosmetology. Volja Publishing company. 2009

Ray Laboratories, Inc. USA. Professional Use Product Manual: Professional Quality Skin Care Product. Version 1.07. Los Angeles, CA 91601. 1-800-525-7292 http://www.rayalab.com/

Wikipedia, Free Encyclopedia. Wikipedia Foundation, Inc, www.en.wikipedia.org.

Online Medical Dictionary at WedMD. 2005-2009 WebMD, LLC. www.webmd.com.

E-zine Articles. www.ezinearticles.com.

Medical Dictionary Online. http://medical-dictionary.com/.